Creative Medical Teaching

About the author

The author is a specialist in the field of medical education. From 1971–1977, he held academic and administrative appointments at the College of Medicine and Dentistry of New Jersey. From 1977–1981, he held successive administrative appointments at South Chicago Community Hospital and the Michael Reese Hospital and Medical Center, both then affiliated with the University of Chicago Pritzker School of Medicine. Since 1981, he has been a faculty member and director of educational development in the Department of Family and Preventive Medicine at the University of Utah School of Medicine.

Neal Whitman has used graduate training in the fields of Higher Education and Health Care Administration to develop methods to improve and evaluate medical teaching. His training in Higher Education was conducted at the University of Michigan (M.A. 1971) and Teachers College, Columbia University (Ed.D. 1979), and his training in Health Care Administration was completed at New York University (M.P.A. 1974).

Dr. Whitman has written over fifty publications and made over fifty presentations at national meetings. He is senior author of *The Chief Resident as Manager* and *Executive Skills for Medical Faculty* as well as the co–author with Dr. Thomas L. Schwenk of *The Physician as Teacher*.

Creative Medical Teaching

Neal Whitman, MPA, Ed.D.
University of Utah School of Medicine

Foreword by Thomas L. Schwenk, M.D.

This book is dedicated to
Elaine Weiss
the most creative teacher I know
and
the best wife I could have.

Contents

Foreword

Thomas L. Schwenk, M.D.
Chairman, Department of Family Practice
University of Michigan School of Medicine

Neal Whitman is a teacher who teaches teachers how to teach. This professional development work can assume the qualities of an Escher print, in which a seemingly hierarchical behavior becomes circular. It is also a high–risk activity, akin to lecturing on the topic of sleep disorders and running the risk of putting the audience to sleep. In this book, Dr. Whitman makes effective use of the circular and systemic attributes of successful teaching, and simultaneously avoids the risk of teaching badly about good teaching. His approach to helping medical teachers become better is novel, entertaining, and scholarly...a combination of adjectives that is too often an oxymoron in the world of educational development.

This book is really a *chrestomathy*. Few readers will know what this is, and fewer still could write one. A chrestomathy is described as "a collection of choice passages from an author, especially one compiled to assist in the acquirement of a language." This book fits both parts of this definition. It contains many choice passages based on Dr. Whitman's extensive professional development experience, and it helps develop a language of excellent teaching. A substantial body of educational research is made useful through Dr. Whitman's wisdom and experience. This statement is not made so much to flatter as to illustrate the critical dilemma in medical education: medical or scientific expertise is a necessary but not sufficient condition for good teaching. Teaching is a process, and, as a profession, is concerned with the domain of relationships, communication, motivation and behavior. Educational research often has little to do with good teaching, and many studies are statistically significant while educationally trivial or unhelpful. I believe this happens because society in general, and the medical profession in particular, values education as an outcome but does not value teaching as a process. When we attempt to value education only as an outcome, we may miss valuable opportunities to understand the teaching processes, interactions, relationships and behaviors that lead to success. Educational outcomes research is important, but only if we understand at a fundamental level the teaching attributes and behaviors which lead to these outcomes. Changes in dependent variables can only be understood if the independent variables are meaningful and are described in sufficient detail.

What does the distinction between process and outcome have to do with this useful book? *Creative Medical Teaching* revels in the process of teaching, and celebrates its importance. By wisely interpreting empirical scholarship, Dr. Whitman provides literally hundreds of tips, tricks and techniques for improving teaching. The format of the book exemplifies Donald Schön's "reflection in action" (1987), with ideas and phrases cross–referenced and linked in a potentially never–ending web of reading to guide the teacher who is making frequent on–the–spot decisions about specific teaching dilemmas. This book should not, and in fact cannot, be read front to back. Similar to our own teaching, it may have a beginning but never has an end. As Dr. Whitman is fond of saying, we have not done our best teaching...yet.

An essay in this book quotes J. Michael Bishop (1984) from the University of California, San Francisco School of Medicine, regarding the purposes of teaching:

> *What are the purposes and priorities of teaching? First, to inspire. Second, to challenge. Third, and only third, to impart information.*

This book meets all three objectives admirably.

How to read this book

     To help you find more than one right answer to the teaching situations you face everyday, this book offers over one hundred topics organized in alphabetical order with cross referencing. So, when I write that "creative teachers are **useful** in what they teach and **novel** in how they teach," the bold lettering lets you know that there are entries for both terms.

     This book is meant for browsing. For example, suppose that you are interested in **clinical teaching**. While perusing this topic, you note the statement, "...**helpful clinical teachers** show interest in clinical care *and* the teaching of it." So, you flip to **Helpful Clinical Teachers**. Three cross–referenced terms in this essay that interest you may be **mentor**, **morning report**, and **preceptor's agenda**. Any one of those terms would lead you to additional reading.

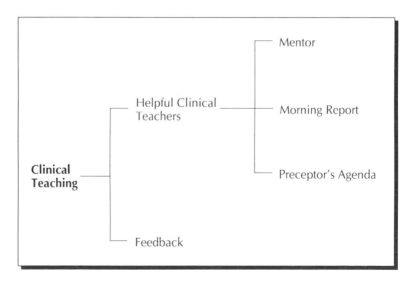

Acknowledgments

An obstacle to the improvement of teaching is that some teachers do not like to be seen "doing it," understandably so. Thus, I would like to thank those individuals at the following client institutions who have allowed me to watch them teach:

Alabama
Carroway Family Medicine Center

California
Fresno Valley Medical Center
Letterman Army Medical Center
University of California, Los Angeles
Veterans Administration Hospital, Los Angeles

Colorado
Fort Collins Family Practice Center
Grand Junction Family Practice Center
Greely Family Practice Center
Mercy Hospital
University of Colorado

Connecticut
Bridgeport Hospital

Hawaii
Tripler Army Medical Center

Illinois
Cook County Hospital
Rush-Presbyterian-St. Luke's Medical Center
St. Francis Medical Center

Indiana
Methodist Hospital

Maryland
Franklin Square Hospital
Johns Hopkins Medical Center
Sinai Hospital
South Baltimore Hospital
Union Memorial Hospital

Massachusetts
Baystate Medical Center
New England College of Optometry

Michigan
Providence Hospital
University of Michigan

Minnesota
Mayo Clinic

Mississippi
Keesler Airforce Medical Center

Missouri
University of Missouri, Kansas City

Montana
Carroll College
University of Montana
Veterans Administration Hospital, Miles City

New Hampshire
Dartmouth Medical School

New York
Albert Einstein College of Medicine
Harlem Hospital
Jacobi Hospital
Maimonides Hospital
New York College of Osteopathic Medicine
New York Medical College
St. Luke's-Presbyterian Hospital
State University of New York, Binghamton
State University of New York, Brooklyn
Syracuse University
University of Rochester

North Dakota
University of North Dakota

Ohio
Akron Medical Center
Cleveland Clinic
Northeastern Ohio Universities College of Medicine
Ohio University College of Osteopathic Medicine

Oklahoma
University of Oklahoma

Pennsylvania
Harrisburg Hospital
Hershey Medical Center

Texas
Baylor Medical College
Texas Tech University
University of Texas, Houston

Tennessee
Vanderbilt University

Utah
Salt Lake Community College
Weber State College

Washington
Madigan Army Medical Center

Washington, D.C.
Walter Reed Army Medical Center

Wyoming
Casper Family Practice Center

Mexico
Autonomous University of Guadalajara

INTRODUCTION

A book is a presumption: it asks for your time and attention, and gives some specks of data, and perhaps amusement (Kappel–Smith 1990).

In asking for your time and attention, I am presuming that you are interested in the improvement of medical teaching. In return, I am offering a data base that draws upon personal experience as well as published research. I hope that you find some amusement in this book. As will be explained later, my purpose is to inspire rather than instruct. My major aim is to encourage creativity in medical teaching.

In 1953 Alan Gregg, a pioneer in medical education, wrote an essay on "Creativeness in Medicine" in which he stated that, "He teaches best who shows his students, not what to think, but how to think…in that long stretch of days awaiting you till, let us say, the year 2000." Thirty years later, the Association of American Medical Colleges published *Physicians for the Twenty–First Century* in which the project panel concluded that medical students should be prepared to learn throughout their professional lives rather than simply to master current information. Lloyd H. Smith, one of the project panel members, entitled his Alan Gregg Memorial Lecture, delivered at the 1984 AAMC Annual Meeting, "Medical Education for the 21st Century." He concluded that, "Medical education must teach the skills for sustained scholarship, or it will fail, no matter how successfully the current state of the art is espoused."

Unfortunately, although there is much talk about training physicians for the twenty–first century, like the weather, little is done about it. The purpose of this book is to help medical teachers show their medical students and residents how to learn, not what to think. In 1953, Gregg called for creativity in medicine. My aim in 1990 is to promote creativity in medical teaching.

Fortunately, whether or not today's medical teachers strive to be more creative, tomorrow's medical teachers may achieve creativity because of changes in the educational system. In "Future–Bound: Glimpses of Life in the 21st Century," Kravitz predicted that education will become more creative because, with home computers linked to computerized libraries, students will be able to explore what they want, when they want. Some medical school freshmen are already more computer–literate than their faculty, which may stimulate these teachers to re–examine their educational methods.

It is not news to today's medical teacher that the information management needs of students are increasing because of an ever–increasing information overload. Anderson and Graham have estimated that medical students must acquire nearly 50,000 facts during the first two years of medical school...a rate of 24 facts for every working hour! It also is not news to today's medical teacher that information is not equal to knowledge. As described by Roszak, knowledge is created by individual minds, drawing on individual experience, separating the significant from the irrelevant, making value judgments. This becomes all too obvious during morning report when a medical student makes a rambling, lengthy case presentation. It is only when the medical student puts together selected patient facts in an organized way that we say he* *knows* the patient.

This book proposes that the challenge for medical education is to help medical students and residents learn how to acquire information and knowledge. In order to become well–informed and knowledgeable, they will have to *learn to learn*, or as stated by Alan Gregg, we have to show

It should be noted at this point that readers are both male and female, of course, but the text consistently uses the pronoun he (or his). Although the s/he construction may reduce gender bias, I feel that it makes awkward reading. My intention is not to promote sex stereotyping, but simply to provide concise writing.

them how to learn, not what to think. To help meet this challenge, this book will encourage medical teachers to be more creative. I am optimistic in the potential of teachers to increase their creativity. The fact that you can read this sentence tells me that already you're using 20 billion brain cells in a complicated way. Everyone is creative, but some people don't let new ideas surface: "The fact that you can walk and talk means you can do 99 percent of what people such as Beethoven and Shakespeare did" (Minsky 1985).

Roger von Oech (1983), a consultant to business and industry, tells his clients that if they want to become more creative, they should believe in the worth of their ideas and have the persistence to keep building on them. He suggests that people look for more than one right answer. Perhaps, if you want to be creative, you must suppress your internal critics for at least one minute. Studies show that when people are asked simply to *pretend that they are creative*, they generate more creative solutions to problems (Stein 1974).

The key to creative teaching lies in finding the second right answer, and the third, and the fourth, and so on. To help you find more than one right answer to teaching situations you face every day, this book will offer you inquiries and investigations, stories and sketches. They are organized in alphabetical order with cross referencing. So, when I write that creative teachers are both **novel** and **useful**, the bold lettering lets you know that there are entries for both terms.

By *novelty* in teaching, I mean using any methods and techniques which help create interest in the learner. **Learning** can be thought of as the acquisition of information and knowledge, but before it can take place, there must be interest. In order to acquire and remember something new, it must stimulate your curiosity in the first place. Learning is the process of **remembering** what you are interested in, and learning and remembering go hand in hand with communication. The most effective communicators are those who understand the role interest plays in the successful delivery of messages (Wurman 1989). This is true for clinicians communicating with patients and for clinical teachers communicating with medical students and residents. Teachers who use novelty help motivate learners and create interest. Novel teaching produces "aha"s and stimulates both the teacher and the learner.

By *useful* teaching, I mean that what is taught is correct, up–to–date, and, most important of all, is relevant to the needs of the learner. All teachers recognize that what they teach must be correct and up–to–date. However, some teachers show little regard for the interests or needs of the learners. For example, a young cardiologist who has joined the staff of a hospital has been asked to speak at Medicine Grand Rounds. He might choose to transmit as much highly complex information as possible within the time allowed in order to validate his professional competence. The teaching would be more useful if, taking into account the needs of the audience members, the cardiologist presented less information, some of which would be useful immediately in their practices (Bunnell 1980).

Creative teachers are novel and useful. Teachers who are novel, but not useful, are charlatans. Those who are useful, but not novel, are pedantic bores. To medical faculty who say to me, "Look, Neal. I'm a teacher, not an entertainer!" I respond, "Let's make a deal. I won't defend the

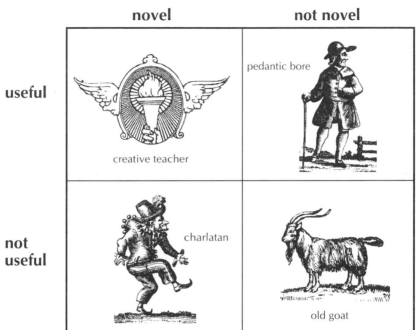

	novel	not novel
useful	creative teacher	pedantic bore
not useful	charlatan	old goat

charlatans if you won't defend the pedantic bores. Can't a teacher be novel *and* useful?"

Creativity is common to both the *practice* of medicine and the *teaching* of medicine. In medicine, a clinician could be said to be creative if he has (a) knowledge and experience, (b) fine judgment, (c) the wisdom to know when conventional thinking is right or wrong, (d) insight to seek options, and (e) imagination to find them (Papper 1984). The same process applies to teaching. In other words, a clinical teacher could be said to be creative if he approaches medical students and residents like his patients. In a sense, both clinical care and clinical teaching have therapeutic goals, *i.e.*, another person is meant to benefit from your encounter. So, just as clinicians diagnose before they treat, clinical teachers should assess before they teach. To those readers who are basic scientists, let me add that the scientific process of hypothesis formulation and testing also is parallel with the teaching process. Furthermore, the creativity essential to quality research is similar to the creativity essential to quality teaching.

The need for creative medical teaching was highlighted in the final words by Magnan in *147 Practical Tips for Teaching Professors* (1989, p. 44):

> Just as Heraclitus observed that we can't step in the same
> stream twice, we can't teach the same class twice.
> Sometimes our strategies and techniques work wonderfully.
> And sometimes the same strategies and techniques miss.
> We usually search for something different when things don't
> work. But we should also try other ways when we're *successful*.
> Why? To avoid tunnel vision and narrow tracks and old
> routines. And so we never forget that we can't
> teach the same class twice.
> Try something *different!*

Whether you are a clinician or a basic scientist or both, I would like you to share the view of an artist who won first place in an art fair. When the judge gave her the prize, she said, "You know, I didn't submit my best work." This surprised the judge who asked her, "Why not?" She replied, "Because I haven't done it yet!" None of us has done our best teaching...yet.

This book is meant to inspire, not instruct. So each topic is discussed briefly with just enough information to get you thinking about your own teaching. Also, this book is meant for browsing. You can start anywhere and jump from topic to topic. Let's say, for example, that you are intrigued by **Physiology Chicken Coop**. After you read about this experiment, in which a non–expert delivered a physiology lecture, you may wish to turn to **Doctor Fox**, a discussion about the original study in which an actor was introduced to a medical audience as a bogus guest lecturer. Upon discovering that no one detected the lecture for the charade that it was, you might want to look up **lecture**, which in turn could lead you to **teaching award winners**, or **knowledge**, or **techniques**. As you can now see, there are many paths through this book. A **metaphor** for this book is a map. You may choose your own destination and your own route. I hope yours is a scenic one.

ADULT LEARNING PRINCIPLES

Until recently, the term "pedagogy" was used to define the profession of teaching without any reference to age. In the 1960s, Malcolm Knowles introduced the term "andragogy" and sought to establish the case for an important difference between the characteristics of adult and child learning. Now pedagogy (with the same Greek root as pediatrics) is widely accepted as a term to refer to the teaching of children and andragogy to the teaching of adults.

When schoolchildren are given the opportunity to learn without direct adult supervision, sometimes they act like adults. Ironically, when medical students are subjected to an information–based (see **lecture**), externally rewarded (see **student tests**) educational system, perhaps we are treating them like children. Whether or not it is fair to call the occasional negative behaviors of medical students "childish," certainly the manifestations are all too familiar to faculty: cutting classes, sleeping in class, and emphasis on grades ("Will it be on the test?").

Since we want to produce lifelong learners, medical schools should take into account the "adultness" of medical students and residents. Personally, I subscribe to the management philosophy advocated by McGregor that people conform to the expectations of their supervisors. (Theory X managers think people like to do as little work as possible and Theory Y managers think work is as natural as play.) If we treat medical students and residents as if they are committed to becoming the best possible physicians, they behave accordingly. However, my own observation is that we produce so much distress in the formal system of medical education that when physicians enter the informal system of continuing medical education, they seek the least challenging educational experiences (see **stress**).

In a handbook for continuing medical educators, Kevin Bunnell proposes five ways in which adults learn. If they have not been turned off by medical school and residency training, these principles will work:

1. Adults usually want to use what they learn soon after they learn it. So, continuing medical education programs should be built on the practice needs of physicians.

2. Adults like to solve problems and not just learn facts (see **problem solving**), so even a lecture should allow time for participation through questions and answers.

3. Learning is best when adults can proceed at their own pace, so independent study should be encouraged.

4. Motivation is increased when adults help set the learning **objectives**, so physicians should be involved in the planning of their own continuing medical education programs. (Alan Knox, a prominent adult educator, once commented that adults like to see themselves as users of, not recipients of, education.)

5. Adults like to know how they are doing, so physicians should be tested on material and given timely **feedback**.

AMBULATORY CARE TRAINING

In 1986, a medical school teacher commented that "teaching clinical medicine in the ambulatory setting is an idea whose time may have finally come" (Perkoff 1986). Yet, a review of the 1986 AAMC survey of senior medical students indicates that 37 percent feel the time devoted to ambulatory care training is insufficient. Interestingly, the figure in 1983 was 35 percent. Other underrepresented topics included care of the elderly, preventive care, and practice management (Gary). So, the time may have come...but not its implementation.

A major obstacle to ambulatory care training is that it is labor intensive. While a hospital attending physician can *concurrently* supervise and teach four students and six residents in a morning rounding session, an attending ambulatory care physician may be able to supervise half that number and typically conducts teaching on a one–to–one basis.

Ambulatory care training occurs in two settings: (1) medical student and resident–staffed clinics with supervising attending physicians and (2) faculty–staffed practices with students and residents serving as **apprentices**. In either setting, there is little time to teach. Reichsman and colleagues called **clinical teaching** "preparedness without preparation" because the instructor has no idea in advance what types of patients will be presented (1964). I liken ambulatory care training to "preparedness without preparation without much time" because the patient in the examination room expects to leave soon.

In resident–staffed clinics, a typical instructor–resident encounter is four minutes, three of which are allocated to the resident's presentation and the attending physician's patient interview. This leaves one minute for teaching! One study suggests that in only one of five cases will the resident and attending physician take the time to see the patient together (Knudson *et al.* 1989).

In faculty–staffed practices, students and residents learn either through observing the faculty or by direct contact with patients that have been delegated to them. If it is a busy practice, little time is available for teaching. Because students can do less, they are expected to observe more than residents do. An irony is that, in many cases, residents can learn more from an observation than a student because they know what to look for and can see subtleties in medical practice.

Because of these time constraints, *negotiation* and *contracting* are critical to making ambulatory care teaching effective. The attending physician and the learner must come to a mutually–understood agreement regarding what the learner can and can not do without supervision. The challenge for the teacher is to allow the learner as much freedom as possible in caring for patients and making decisions without compromising medical care quality. Thus, the little time available for "teaching" must be allocated to assessment, not just instruction. Assessment and instruction comprise the **preceptor's agenda**.

Two excellent ambulatory teachers at the University of Michigan Medical School, James O. Woolliscroft (Internal Medicine) and Thomas L. Schwenk (Family Medicine), have noted six possible educational goals for any ambulatory–based educational experience (1989):

1. *Observation of the Natural or Treated History*
    Following patients through portions or all phases of illness provides a different view of the impact of that disease upon a single patient than can be gained from a hospital experience.

2. *Developing Appropriate Professional Expectations and Attitudes about Chronic Illness*
    The ambulatory setting provides different opportunities than the hospital setting for teaching students about the impact of disease upon patients and family members.

3.   *Social, Financial, and Ethical Aspects of Medical Practice*

Practice issues that frequently confront practicing physicians, but are rarely taught in the medical school, can be addressed in ambulatory care experiences.

4.   *Patient Communication and Negotiation Skills*

The ambulatory care setting is especially well–suited to learning the physician–patient communication skills that are essential to long–term management of patient problems.

5.   *Clinical **Problem Solving***

Ambulatory care problem solving is usually stepwise and more deductive than in the hospital where patients may be admitted for a specific set of tests and discharged.

6.   *Faculty **Role Models***

One–to–one ambulatory care teaching provides an opportunity for developing stronger teacher–learner relationships than possible in a hospital team.

ANECDOTES

Telling an anecdote can be a creative teaching **technique.** For example, a physiology teacher at the University of Michigan Medical School effectively got across the principle that urine is essentially composed, not of waste products, but rather of water and salts which are present in the body in excess, by telling his students about his canoe trip in the wilderness area of Michigan's upper peninsula. Due to the hordes of mosquitoes, he and his wife did not want to leave their tent at night. When nature called, they emptied their bladders in the coffee pot. Knowing there was nothing harmful in urine, except maybe a few bacteria from the urethral orifice that would easily be killed by boiling, they brewed coffee in the morning without worry (Mouw 1981).

Of course, telling an anecdote to make a point is not the same as using personal experiences as substitutes for scientific practice. In fact, with six actual clinical cases, three faculty members at the University of Washington School of Medicine demonstrated that subjective learning can lead to suboptimal clinical **problem solving.** In one case, a resident was ridiculed when he suggested an uncommon diagnosis for a severely ill patient. At exploratory surgery, the resident's diagnosis was found to be correct. He was highly praised, and subsequently overdiagnosed this disease, repeatedly ordering premature consideration of, and testing for, this uncommon diagnosis (Featherstone, Beitman, and Irby 1984).

Medical students and residents should look upon each patient as a learning experience; however, unusual cases can result in learning the wrong lesson. Similarly, medical teachers should be careful when using clinical experiences to make a point that is uncontrolled in a scientific sense. In order to avoid **problem solving biases,** please consider the recommendations of Featherstone and colleagues:

1.   The role of prior experiences in determining medical decisions should be reduced.

2.   Exceptionally successful or unfavorable outcomes should be viewed as chance–related events.

3.   Causal relationships between case outcomes and behaviors of doctors should be de–emphasized, especially in a judgmental sense.

4.   Unusual anecdotes should serve as a stimulus to introduce the scientific method into the subjective learning process of medical education.

5.   A more systemized, unbiased way of using prior experiences to improve medical care should be devised; for example, using computers to record patient conditions, prognostic factors, and outcomes.

APPRENTICESHIP

In *The Physician as Teacher*, Schwenk and Whitman (1987) devote a chapter to teaching ambulatory medicine. Undoubtedly, **ambulatory care training** is becoming an important component of medical education. The reasons for this are complex and include the fewer inpatients available for teaching due to a decreased number of hospital admissions and shorter lengths of stay. The shift from inpatient to outpatient teaching has spilled out of the teaching hospital into private practices for reasons equally complex, including the need for additional medical teachers. Many of these **preceptorships** are staffed by voluntary faculty.

Teaching medical students outpatient medicine in a private practice is not a new idea. In fact, in the pre–Flexner days and before the advent of the modern teaching hospital, most medical teaching occurred at the side of private practitioners. Because I believe that teaching by private doctors will increase, I prefer to call this "the return of the apprentice." The desirability of teaching clinical medicine in the private office was highlighted by one medical school faculty member who commented, "Learning primary care in a university hospital is like trying to learn forestry in a lumber-yard" (Verby *et al.* 1981). This dichotomy between what is taught versus what is practiced also was noted by the *GPEP Physicians for the Twenty–First Century* report: "Although fewer than five percent of all physician/patient contacts results in hospitalization, clinical clerkships are predomi-nantly based on hospital inpatient services" (1984).

At a national meeting convened to discuss the GPEP report, one first–year resident described her feelings of inadequacy in the ambulatory care setting:

> During my first afternoon in the clinic, my deficiencies in outpatient–based medicine became all too apparent when faced with my first patient, a 55–year–old female with three volumes of old charts.... She had come in to meet her doctor, and I had a one–hour appointment during which to evaluate her complaints of palpitations, dizziness, dysuria, and confusion over the nine different medicines she reported taking each day. I panicked because I did not know how to (a) structure my agenda for working with her medical problems, (b) take care of acute problems while working with an incomplete data base, and (c) develop the beginning of our three–year relationship, all within one hour (Mangione, p. 3).

I believe that medical students will be better prepared for residency training and residents will be better prepared for practice if more teaching occurs in a medical practice at the side of a private physician. This does not mean a return to the pre–Flexner era of medical education. Today's preceptorship represents a union of academic medicine and the ongoing practice of medicine and serves to bring the medical school closer to the communities that support the school and consume its services and products (Bishop 1987).

ARTIFICIAL REALITY

First meetings between computers and humans often resemble awkward early sex. You don't know where to put your hands or how to ask for what you want. The basic instructions you were given don't seem to fit this particular case, and you're afraid of doing some damage. Most certainly you will make mistakes and, if your fear is great enough, you might not able to do anything at all. And so the first time you interact with this new partner, you're likely to experience a lot of anxiety (Gabgan 1983).

Certainly, there are many uses for the computer in medical education (D. Swanson 1984):

1. Drill and practice presents a succession of exercise questions designed to provide practice in a particular subject area, for example, calculating drug dosages.

2. A tutorial is similar to a programmed text in which the student is led through the material via a structured question and answer dialogue, for example reading ECGs.

3. A **simulation** models a real life situation. For example, the Iliad program at the University of Utah School of Medicine creates a patient problem. The student elicits data and makes a differential diagnosis.

4. Computer–based testing provides immediate scoring and feedback.

5. Computer–managed instruction assists students and teachers by tracking material covered, tests taken, assignments completed, *etc.*

The newest breakthrough in medical computing is "artificial reality," the ability to program a custom universe in a computer. Perhaps the best known example of artificial reality is the flight simulator used to train pilots. In training surgeons to perform rhinoplasty, for example, a computer program that simulates bone, cartilage, and skin could help residents analyze each move, reversing incisions to create the best results. As explained by Dr. Bill Morain, professor of plastic surgery at Dartmouth, it would be better to learn first via the computer than by doing 500 nose jobs and screwing up 400 of them (Nash 1990).

ATTENTION SPAN

A boring teacher is someone who talks in someone else's sleep.

Maintaining an audience's attention is a challenge. This was illustrated by H.G. Frost's observations of the presidential address at the annual meeting of the British Association for the Advancement of Science. Frost noted that the speaker, while not in the class of Sir John Gielgud, was adequate. Nevertheless, he had difficulty holding the audience's attention (1965):

9:03   Speaker starts.

9:12   My attention has wandered. Some people have closed eyes.

9:18   About ten percent in view show signs of attention wandering.

9:20   Perhaps one–third of audience fidgeting and ten percent on the platform.

9:22   Impossible to keep my eye on all the fidgeting on the platform.

9:28   People looking at their programs. Two look at their watches.

9:30   Hard to make myself concentrate for a whole paragraph.

9:38   Everybody in sight has now let attention wander.

9:42   Whispered conversation on the platform.

9:43   Nobody I watch seems to concentrate for many minutes.

9:46   Speaker refers to world population and food problem: general alertness.

9:48   Alertness passes. Trance more noticeable than fidgeting.

9:49   Speaker makes small joke. Only a feeble twitter. Some very delayed smiles on the platform.

9:50   One or two really asleep. One man reads a newspaper, I think.

9:52   Unless I concentrate very hard it sounds like a stream of platitudes.

9:56   End. Applause.

Studies of attention span, including one study of medical students, show that **student concentration**, on the average, rises to a maximum at ten to fifteen minutes and then falls steadily until the end of a lecture.

ATTITUDINAL CHANGE

Wissen macht frei (knowledge liberates).

Goethe summed up the challenge of education when he stated, "Knowing is not enough; we must apply. Willing is not enough; we must do." Implicit in this statement is the understanding that having the right attitude also is important. Why is it, then, that educators typically emphasize the **knowledge** and **skills** they intend to teach, and rarely specify attitudinal change? A visiting medical teacher from Sweden told me that in German there is a distinction made between *wissen,* meaning "knowing what," and *konnen,* meaning "knowing how." But, as far as he knew, there was not a German word for "knowing why." Yet most students want to know why something is to be learned before they learn it.

It is much more difficult to influence a change in attitude than a change in knowledge and skills. However, attitudinal change is essential to educating the kinds of physicians we want. An attitude may be a primary **objective** of instruction; for example, influencing our trainees to believe that all patients deserve to be treated with respect. Other attitudes may be secondary objectives, *i.e.,* as a prerequisite to learning new knowledge. For example, how attentive will a medical student be to a lecture on the diagnosis and treatment of alcoholism if he feels that treating alcoholic patients is a waste of time? Stanford Erickson, who directed the University of Michigan's Center for Research on Learning and Teaching, stated that, "Most instruction involves a two–part process: presenting information while at the same time indicating its worth" (p. 5).

To highlight the importance of attitude to learning new knowledge and skills, I often ask medical teachers if they have children. If they do, I ask whether their children do all the things they know they should do and know how to do. As you can imagine, the answer almost always is, "No, not all the time." Then I ask, "Why not?" Usually, the explanation has something to do with "attitude." This comparison of parenting to teaching was first made by Gordon who applied the principles of *Parent Effectiveness Training* to *Teacher Effectiveness Training* and, in both books, recommended active listening to the *emotional* as well as factual contents of a message.

In a guide to clinical teaching, it is recommended that preceptors assess prior to instruction (Whitman and Schwenk, 1984). In other words, before reinforcing good attitudes or modifying bad attitudes, it is essential to discover current attitudes. The assessment of their attitudes is really an assessment of their budding professional behaviors. Of course, we can never *really* know another person's attitudes except as these are demonstrated through behavior. The challenge for a clinical teacher is to look and listen in a manner that will give you the best opportunity of seeing your learner's behavior clearly and accurately.

You probably are aware that medical students may say and do things to portray attitudes which they think you support. This attempt to mask real attitudes is not new to physicians. Their patients may do this as well. Sometimes patients do this when their physician tries to promote a life style change. Students and residents share with patients the desire to make a good impression. Uncovering their true attitudes requires some creativity.

Based on suggestions for clinical teachers generated by Stritter *et al.* (1975), Irby (1978), and Lamkin *et al.* (1983), five approaches can be used to discern learner attitudes:

1.   Develop *rapport* with students and residents by sharing your own personal feelings.

2.   Show genuine *interest* in learners by treating them as colleagues.

3.   Be *accessible* to them by being patient with them and recognizing the extra time it takes to teach on a one–to–one basis.

4.   Be *empathic* by remembering what it was like to be a student or a resident.

5.   Be *non–judgmental* by acknowledging differences among people.

Dr. Schwenk and I use the term "professional intimacy" to sum up these five approaches. What is being suggested here is that by being yourself you can encourage students and residents to be themselves. We recommend that you treat your learners the way you treat your patients.

If you are successful in assessing the current attitudes of students and residents, there will be many positive attitudes that you want to reinforce. This is the easy and fun part of clinical teaching. But what do you do when the attitudes you uncover are not the ones you want developed in future physicians? As Gordon pointed out in *Parent Effectiveness Training*, moralizing and preaching probably will not work. In fact, using moral, ethical, or professional failure to stimulate guilt in medical students or residents may only encourage covert behavior or passive resistance.

Since you cannot *tell* someone else how to be, consider *showing* them how to be and, by your example, make being that way seem desirable and worthwhile. In other words, use creative approaches to be a **role model**. Be explicit and honest about how you deal with the uncertainties, difficulties, and ambiguities of medical practice. Avoid playing the **pretend to know game**. Discuss how you cope with **stress**. Reveal how you handle difficult patient encounters. In promoting attitudinal change, please keep in mind the advice of Herman Hesse in *Magister Ludi*, "Truth is lived, not taught."

BAD TEACHING

Those who can do; those who cannot, teach.
Those who cannot teach, administer.
Those who cannot administer, consult.

According to Mark E. Saul, a winner of the National Science Foundation Presidential Award in 1984 for excellence in teaching, bad teaching is learned in colleges and universities where good teaching is neither fostered nor rewarded. The problem there may be due to the belief that teaching is not doing. George Bernard Shaw formulated this common suspicion about teachers: "He who can does; he who cannot teaches." Yet, as Professor Saul points out, "Not every scholar can keep up with developments in his or her field, maintain an enthusiastic attitude toward learning and inspire others with that enthusiasm. *Those who can, teach* (1988)."

The late Kenneth Eble, an award–winning professor at the University of Utah, also blamed bad teaching on the belief that teaching was not, in itself, "doing." He felt that teaching is doing of a very important kind: "If teachers would develop a respect for their craft, they must begin by acknowledging that what a teacher 'does' matters and proceed by developing skill in the many things teachers do" (1988, p.12).

The belief that teaching is not doing is one of the **myths of teaching**.

BEDSIDE TEACHING

Clinical faculty may do less bedside teaching than they think. According to a study in one teaching hospital, attending physicians spent only 16 percent of rounding time at the bedside and, for half that time, the patient was not necessary to the discussion. Yet, bedside teaching is considered by many the essence of medical training (Collins *et al.* 1978).

Can you imagine medical education without bedside teaching? I would presume not. In fact, learning the "healing art" by examining sick and injured people probably can be traced to prehistoric cave dwellers. In a tradition dating back to the Middle Ages, European doctors believed that medicine was a suitable subject for university instruction, and bedside teaching was conducted by university teachers. This practice continued into the Renaissance. Perhaps the most famous clinical teacher of the seventeenth century was Franciscus de la Boe Sylvius, who is remembered today for brain structures that bear his name: aqueduct of Sylvius and the sylvian fissure. As the chairman of Medicine at Leiden, he developed a medical teaching method relevant today:

> My method (is to) lead my students by hand to the practice of medicine, taking them everyday to see patients in the public hospital, that they may hear the patients' symptoms and see their physical findings. Then I question the students as to what they have noted in the patients and about their thoughts and perceptions regarding the causes of the illness and the principles of treatment (Linfors and Neelson 1980, p. 1231).

Until the twentieth century, it was not clear that university–trained doctors were more effective than those who learned by **apprenticeship** at the side of a local practitioner. In any case, whether aspiring physicians learned from university teachers or from local practitioners, most medical training occurred at the bedside. Because training in a medical school had questionable benefit, most American doctors in eighteenth century America learned by apprenticeship. This apprentice system was "based upon empiricism and magic, supplemented now and then by a little science" (Miller 1962, p. 104).

In his commencement address at the Medical College of Philadelphia in 1765, Dr. John Morgan proposed that medical education be based on a broad premedical education, a fundamental science program, and clinical training at the bedside of patients in an affiliated college. However, until a true scientific foundation was laid, implementation of that model was limited. Looking at American medical schools a hundred years later, medical education was hopelessly unscientific and ineffective.

However, with the founding of the Johns Hopkins Medical School in 1893, the entire situation was transformed. A revolution in academic medicine was based on the German university model, which linked teaching to research. Scientific breakthroughs in the field of biology made science highly relevant to medical practice, and bedside teaching at the medical school became a teaching **method** with more substance. The Flexner Report of 1910 validated this linkage between medical knowledge and bedside teaching.

A primary advocate of bedside teaching during this revolution in medical education was William Osler, Professor of Medicine at Johns Hopkins:

> How can we make the work of the student in
> the third and fourth year...practical...? The

answer is, take him from the lecture room, take him from the amphitheater—put him in the outpatient department—put him in the wards (1903, p. 49).

Dr. Henry A. Christian relived the days fifty years earlier, when he learned at the bedside with Osler:

> The discussions seemed very informal, possibly a bit haphazard; yet a surprisingly complete description of the patient and his disease was left with the students.... His criticism of students and their work were incisive and unforgettable, but never harsh or unkindly; they inspired respect and affection, never fear (1949, p. 82).

A second revolution in Medicine followed World War II. The explosion of knowledge and the pervasiveness of specialization has made medicine highly technological. Some medical educators believe that these factors have led to negligence in bedside teaching. For example, one member of the Department of Internal Medicine at the University of Michigan complained that many colleagues were reluctant to teach medical students the basic skills of taking a patient's history and performing a physical examination at the bedside:

> Professors are in the main eager to lecture to whole classes on the most modern advances in medical practice, but eschew the opportunity to make a more lasting impression on the practice of medicine by helping the same students to attain competence in clinical skills (Sisson 1976, p. 145).

The de–emphasis on teaching clinical skills at the bedside was noted by Dr. Ludwig W. **Eichna**, who completed four years of medical school after retiring from the chairmanship of the Department of Medicine at the State University of New York–Downstate Medical Center. Eichna complained that clinical skills were not adequately taught and that both housestaff and students focused on the "numbers" rather than on the patient. He asked, "Shall future medicine see the replacement of clinical skills by technologic procedures" (1980, p. 731)?

In a similar vein, Drs. Linfors and Neelson at the Duke Medical Center wrote an editorial in *The New England Journal of Medicine* that stated, "A return to the bedside provides an opportunity (although the teacher may not act on it) to encourage and exemplify attitudes and values of enduring worth to the student and the patient" (1980 p. 1233). See **attitudinal change**.

In reaction to this editorial, Dr. S. Roger Hirsch responded that, having made Internal Medicine rounds for the past twenty years, he has noticed that during the past five years there has been a "steady progression toward leaving the bedside and congregating around the **coffee cup**, preferably in front of a blackboard" (1981, p. 738). One of the other respondents, Dr. Henry S. Kahn, from the Emory University School of Medicine, wrote that more teaching was needed in the ambulatory setting as well as the hospital bedside—a position fully supported by Linfors and Neelson who replied that, "We prefer a **metaphorical** interpretation of the bedside to include all learning that incorporates the patient's presence and focuses on the patient—whether in the hospital, the home, or the clinician's office" (1981, p. 738).

For clinical teachers who wish to improve their teaching skills in the inpatient or ambulatory care setting, two resources are the chapter on bedside teaching in *The Physician as Teacher* (Schwenk and Whitman 1987) and *Teaching During Attending Rounds* (Weinholtz 1987).

Schwenk and Whitman recommend that the bedside teacher should:

1. Base all teaching on data generated by or about the patient.

2. Conduct bedside rounds with respect for the patient's dignity.

3. Use bedside teaching particularly for teaching psychomotor **skills**.

4. Use every opportunity in bedside teaching to provide **feedback** to learners.

According to Weinholtz, the challenge of simultaneously addressing the patient's emotional needs and the team's learning needs makes bedside teaching a delicate exercise. He recommends that the bedside teacher:

1. Try to avoid having team members present cases to you in front of the patient or using bedside visits strictly for collecting information for your own benefit.

2. When possible, actively demonstrate to team members ways of discovering physical findings.

3. Observe team members' efforts to discover these findings; reinforce their efforts and engage them in non–threatening discussion about findings.

4. Do not require the entire team to visit all patients during rounds. Instead, have team members visit their own patients and selected patients from whom they might learn a great deal.

5. When possible, alert team members beforehand to behaviors that you want to demonstrate at the bedside. If no forewarning can be given, be sure to address your behavior in follow–up discussions.

BORING TEACHERS

Good teaching cannot be equated with technique. It comes from the integrity of the teacher, from his or her relation to subject and students, from the capricious chemistry of it all. A method that lights one class afire extinguishes another. An approach that bores one student changes another's life (Palmer 1990, p. 11).

Carl Rogers, the pioneer of indirect counseling, has claimed that one person cannot teach another how to teach (1969). I disagree. I think I can teach a teacher how to create an environment in which learning is facilitated. What does such an environment look like? First and foremost, the teacher has the learner's attention (see **attention span**). You cannot hold a student's attention if you lack **enthusiasm** or are boring. According to the social psychologist, Mark R. Leary (1986), the degree of boredom is equivalent to the amount of effort one must exert in order to pay attention to something. Students become bored when teachers show little emotion and are tedious. By little emotion I mean talking in a monotonous voice, showing little facial expression, and maintaining little eye contact. By tedious I mean talking too slowly, taking five minutes to make a fifteen–second point, and digressing from the main point. These boring behaviors can be changed. Teachers who are boring can learn not to be.

Of course, some people blame their subject matter rather than themselves. My view is that people are boring, not subjects. I agree with the late poet, John Ciardi, who said that there were no boring teachers, only boring people in classrooms impersonating teachers. I call these impersonators "pedantic bores." Pedantic bores may be **useful** in what they teach, but not **novel** in how they teach it. On the other hand, some teachers are novel, but not useful. I call these people "charlatans." Being useful in what you teach requires more than being correct and up–to–date. It also requires being relevant. Relevance means teaching at the students' level, using examples and even **metaphors** to make the material understandable and memorable. Students can tell whether or not their teachers care that the subject is learned.

The imagination needed to be creative was described by Jacob Bronowski (1978):

> If science is a form of imagination, if all experiment is a form of play, then science cannot be dry–as–dust. Yet many people suppose it is; this is a popular fallacy, that art is fun but science is dull.
>
> Neither art nor science is dull; no imaginative activity is dull to those who are willing to reimagine it for themselves. Of course, many individual scientists are personally dull; but I assure you, after a lifetime of suffering both, that many artists are dull people too. But they are not dull inside their work—neither the artists nor the scientists. Inside their work they are at play, they are imagining and creating new situations, and that is the greatest fun in the world for them—and for us, if we can recreate their work.
>
> Science or art, every creative activity is fun. But no creative work, in art or science, truly exists for us unless we ourselves help recreate it.

BRAINSTORMING

Brainstorming is probably the best known and most widely used **technique** for stimulating creativity (Stein 1975). The brainstorming technique was developed by an advertising executive, Alex F. Osborn, in response to his dissatisfaction with the "usual" business meeting. To generate a wide variety of creative ideas in a short amount of time, Osborn asked participants to refrain from judgment and to abstain from working on any single idea too long. He called these sessions "brainstorming" because people were asked to "use the brain to storm a problem."

According to Osborn (1963), there are two kinds of thinking: the judicial mind and the creative mind. The *judicial* mind "analyzes, compares, and chooses," whereas the *creative* mind "visualizes, foresees and generates ideas." Today we associate those two kinds of thinking with the left brain hemisphere which is intellectual and excels in analysis and synthesis (judicial) and the right brain hemisphere which is intuitive and operates holistically (creative). The judicial mind "puts the brakes" on the creative mind, and the aim of brainstorming is to remove these brakes so that ideas can be generated. Thus, one principle of brainstorming is *deferred judgment*. Participants should be encouraged to volunteer ideas without concern for their value, feasibility, or significance, all of which can be considered later. A second principle of brainstorming is that *quantity breeds quality*. Since our first ideas may be the "safest," it is necessary to "get through" these if we are to arrive at the more original ones (Stein).

There are four basic rules in conducting a brainstorming session:

1.   Rule out criticism.

2.   Welcome freewheeling.

3.   Push for quantity.

4.   Seek combination and improvement.

When you use this technique, anticipate that students and residents are accustomed to being evaluated for their responses to questions and are conditioned to be concrete. As a result, they may have trouble volunteering their ideas in the freewheeling, non–judgmental atmosphere of a brainstorming session. These obstacles also occur in workshops I conduct for medical faculty. I must be prepared to explain the purpose of brainstorming and to be encouraging. When I conduct a workshop on the techniques of teaching, I sometimes ask the participants to brainstorm the question, "Why might the **coffee cup** be my favorite teaching tool?" My aim is to discover whether they already understand the need for teachers to stop, look and listen.

CLINICAL IMPRESSIONS

A medical student asked his attending physician how one acquires good clinical judgment. The response was, "from experience." Then the student asked how to acquire experience. The response was, "from bad clinical judgment."

In a letter to the editor of *The Journal of Medical Education* (1987), Drs. Ellen and William Crain asked others to join in the study of clinical impressions so that clinical judgment could be taught. They had already asked five highly regarded attending pediatricians, nine second and third year pediatric residents, and thirteen pediatric interns to report their thoughts and feelings as they examined children under the age of two with fever. Analysis of the tape–recorded examinations showed that residents and interns observed the children in a detached manner, whereas the attending physicians made special efforts to get a personal sense of the children. These attendings explained, for the benefit of the housestaff, that if one talks gently and respectfully to even young infants, these patients will react in ways which will indicate how sick or well they are feeling.

While the Crains believe that there is too much emphasis on rational mental processes in the study of medical **problem solving**, colleagues and I have argued that asking clinicians to report their thoughts and feelings during patient evaluations will emphasize rational mental processes...appropriately so! We believe that clinical impressions are rational, but may be automatic (Whitman *et al.* 1988). Automatic mental processes are activated at *unconscious* levels, allowing an experienced clinician to make conclusions quickly while relying upon intuition and insight. In contrast, less experienced medical students and residents use controlled mental processes which are activated at *conscious* levels. They follow set guidelines step–by–step when confronted by a patient's symptoms.

Both unconscious and conscious mental processes are rational. What differs is how the person knows that something is so. Donald Schön (1987) speaks of knowing more than one can say. Clinical impression is an example of "knowing–in–action." The knowing is in the action and is revealed by spontaneous and skillful execution. Yet, it may be difficult to explain one's own actions. When the medical teacher is unconsciously competent, he may find it difficult to articulate his thinking to a medical student or resident (see **skills**).

The "think aloud" protocol, advocated by Ellen and William Crain, provides an effective **technique** for teaching clinical impressions to medical students and residents. Another solution lies in the computer. The Department of Internal Medicine and the Department of Medical Informatics at the University of Utah School of Medicine are implementing a computer program named "Iliad," which elicits data for an actual patient being seen by a third–year medical student. For each datum, Iliad can reveal its information value and identify what pathophysiological processes it "has in mind." Of course, the computer's "mind" is not a black box, but a set of rational constructs elicited from experienced clinicians and culled from the literature. Whereas the individual clinical teacher may be unconsciously competent, the aggregate thinking expressed in Iliad will exhibit conscious competence, thus supplementing the student's education.

CLINICAL PERFORMANCE TESTING

Clinical teachers are faced with the difficult task of measuring cognitive, affective, and psychomotor **objectives** which are being performed simultaneously. Four tools can help test clinical performance (Whitman 1982):

1. *Checklists* provide a breakdown of performance into specific steps as well as a list of common errors, making documentation less time–consuming. According to Irby and Dohner (1976), there are seven characteristics of effective checklists:
    a. clear instructions
    b. behaviorally stated terms
    c. only critical items included
    d. option for "not observed" category
    e. objective criteria
    f. instructional objectives reflected
    g. items arranged in natural order of sequence for performing the skill

2. *Observation logs* allow each objective to be pre–printed with additional space for writing notes. Whereas a checklist pre–establishes what to note, an

observation log provides an opportunity to assess more complex skills in an open–ended format (Knopke and Diekelman 1978).

3.   *Critical incident forms* are used to identify a critical aspect of performance, positive or negative, which can be pre–printed. When something noteworthy has been witnessed, the evaluator documents what happened on the critical incident form (Ingalsbe and Spears 1979).

4.   *Anecdotal records* provide a place to write brief descriptions of any situations which seem relevant to the evaluation of clinical performance.

What all four tools have in common is that evaluation is concurrent with performance, *i.e.*, data are collected and recorded at the same time that the student is performing. In contrast, student rating forms are completed at the end of a clinical rotation. When there is no evaluation until the end, we are relying on only our recall. The key to effective **student evaluation** is using multiple methods of data collection (Guba and Lincoln 1981).

CLINICAL TEACHING

Clinical teaching "is unique in the entire realm of teaching. In no other field does the nature of the material demand of the teacher this degree of preparedness without preparation" (Reichsman *et al.* 1964).

The fact that the clinical teacher does not know ahead of time the "topic" to be taught underscores the importance of *process* skills that will produce "helpful interactions" between the teacher and the learner (Skeff *et al.* 1984). For example, the teacher should communicate educational goals at the start, give **feedback** along the way, and provide an evaluation at the end. Also, it is helpful to establish a challenging, but not threatening, learning environment (see **stress**) and to focus attention on **knowledge, attitudinal change**, and **skills**. Finally, it is critical that the clinical teacher promote understanding and continued self–learning.

Clinical teachers may know more about these helpful interactions than they think because of their experience with employer–employee, parent–child, and physician–patient relationships. As employers, clinicians may have learned Blanchard and Johnson's three secrets of management: one minute goals, praisings, and reprimands (1982). As parents, clinicians may have learned Gordon's two rules of parent effectiveness: listen to the factual and emotional level and, whenever possible, negotiate win–win solutions (1970). As physicians, clinicians may have learned Dodge's physician–patient exchanges: information, emotion, and meaning (1983).

The importance of process skills was further underscored by a survey of third and fourth year medical students which asked them to identify helpful clinical teaching behaviors (Stritter, Hain, and Grimes 1975). According to these students, **helpful clinical teachers** show interest in clinical care *and* in the teaching of it. They explain what they are thinking and doing. In addition, they involve students in the process of **problem solving**.

CLINICAL TEACHING IS LIKE CLINICAL CARE

Clinical teaching is like clinical care in that both use the same set of interactive communication skills (see **PAP Smear**). For example, during *attentive silence*, clinicians assume low control over the interaction and provide the patient with high control. Clinical teachers use these same skills when they want to assess the learner's needs so that they can target instruction (see **preceptor's agenda**). They use a set of skills contained in *cooperative negotiation* with patients when they establish two–way communication. Clinical teachers use these same skills when they want to share experiences and promote **problem solving**. Finally, sometimes clinicians use the art of *persuasion* with patients. In a similar fashion, clinical teachers may wish to correct or challenge the thinking of a student or resident.

Thus, through attentive silence, cooperative negotiation, and persuasion, clinical teachers use all the communication skills they already have developed as clinicians. Effective **clinical teaching** is a matter of providing helpful interactions rather than presenting a specific body of information.

Effective clinical teachers often look like accordion players. First, they open up the conversation with open–ended questions. Then, they close in with more specific questions. When they sense that they have learned enough for the time being, they open up the conversation again. These teachers are using the same skills they use as clinicians. As clinicians, they first ask their patients open–ended questions such as, "What brought you here today?" Then, they focus on one or two issues before opening up the conversation again by asking, "Is there anything else on your mind?" As clinical teachers, they might ask for a student's differential diagnosis, focus on one or two hypotheses and then return to broader issues.

Clinicians frequently see patients under constraining conditions. There may be little time and few support services. "Cure" may not be a realistic objective. Yet, they still try to be "therapeutic" in the sense of being helpful to another person. What might be helpful may be as little as providing reassurance or answering a question. Yet, the same clinicians may feel frustrated when there is little time to teach and few educational support services. Rather than "teaching it all" (the educational equivalent of "cure"), clinical teachers could aim at more realistic objectives such as providing reassurance or answering a question!

Stuart and Lieberman (1986) believe that every clinician who can communicate with patients has the basic tools to provide basic counseling. My premise is that, in addition, every clinician with those basic interactive skills also knows how to teach. Just as talking with a patient is primarily a theme–centered conversation based on the patient's concerns, teaching a medical student or resident is a theme–centered conversation based on the student's learning needs.

CLINICAL TEACHING STYLES

Family Medicine educators at the University of Massachusetts adapted a classification scheme developed in a study of physicians and their patients to identify four styles in the faculty–resident relationship (Bibace *et al.* 1981):

1. *Assertive Style*
    Gives directions.
    Asks questions.
    Gives information.
    Asks self–answering questions.

2. *Suggestive Style*
    Offers opinion.
    Suggests with questions.
    Suggests with statements.
    Relates personal experience as a model for the learner.

3. *Collaborative Style*
    Elicits learner's ideas.
    Accepts learner's ideas.
    Explores learner's ideas.
    Relates personal experience as a means of empathizing with the learner.

4. *Facilitative Style.*
    Elicits learner's feelings.
    Accepts learner's feelings
    Offers feelings.
    Encourages the learner.

I agree strongly with Bibace and his colleagues that there is no single correct clinical teaching style. The aim should be for clinical teachers to match a teaching style to a resident in a particular situation. For this very reason, I emphasize that medical teaching must include assessment as well as instruction (see **preceptor's agenda**).

COFFEE CUP

When I conduct workshops on **techniques** of teaching, I often begin with a **brainstorming** question: "Why might the coffee cup be my favorite teaching tool?" I discovered this use for a coffee cup from Peter Kugel, an associate professor of computer science at Boston College. He wrote in *The New York Times* about a workshop for new faculty where experienced faculty explained how to use the blackboard, how to show **slides**, how to make up student tests, *etc.* Kugel remembers enjoying their presentations, but not remembering a thing they said.

Then during the coffee break, a mathematics professor mentioned that his favorite teaching tool was "a cup of coffee." The professor explained that he tends to talk too much and too fast in the classroom, so every once in a while, he takes a sip of coffee to slow down the pace and to give the students a chance to think. Kugel began bringing a cup of coffee to class and found that these pauses gave him, as well as the students, time to think. He also discovered that he could use these pauses to look around the room and assess the students' reactions to the class. In other words, he began to evaluate the **teaching–learning process** as it was occurring!

When I brainstorm with the coffee cup question (holding a cup of coffee and pausing after a sip), participants generate many ideas, including:

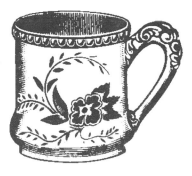

• The coffee wakes you up.

• With a cup of coffee, you set an informal atmosphere.

• It gives people a chance to ask a question.

• It stops you from talking too fast.

• The students will feel free to bring their own cup of coffee.

I was heartened to learn that the brainstorming process continued after a workshop. On August 11, 1989, I used the coffee cup brainstorming question in a workshop for faculty and residents in the Department of Family Medicine at the University of Missouri–Kansas City. In a letter dated August 16, Dr. David Govaker, an assistant professor, wrote to me:

> I had my usual 'breakfast sludge' of yogurt, dried fruit, and bran cereal in the Neal Whitman Memorial Coffee Cup. You should know

that, according to our pilot study, the beneficial effect of the coffee cup is independent of
content. We are considering a placebo–control
trial of 'no cup' versus 'empty cup' versus
'coffee' versus 'breakfast sludge.' If we are able
to obtain funding, I will be sure to include
several site visits for you as a consultant.

CONNOISSEURSHIP

Many creative teachers have developed a "taste" for
good **teaching**, *i.e.*, they have become connoisseurs of teaching. A person can become a connoisseur of almost anything.
I happen to be a connoisseur of Southwestern American
Indian pottery. Basically, a connoisseur is a person with
informed and astute discrimination. When I look at a piece of
pottery I can probably tell you in which pueblo it was made
and whether it is a good or bad example of pottery made
there. In addition, I have formed my own opinions of which
types of pottery I prefer. Thus, there are objective (identify-
ing the pueblo and rating its pottery) and subjective (my
likes and dislikes) aspects of connoisseurship. The same can
be said of teaching. A connoisseur of teaching can identify
the methods and techniques of teaching being used and
evaluate how well these are matched to the instructional
objectives, as well as forming opinions regarding a teacher's
effectiveness.

Elliot Eisner, who began his academic career in art
education and today teaches at the Stanford University
Graduate School of Education, is the most noteworthy
proponent of the "connoisseur in teaching" concept. He says
that educational connoisseurship is the art of knowing and
appreciating what is educationally significant. To become a
connoisseur of anything requires experience. For example, as
Eisner points out, to become a connoisseur of wine, one

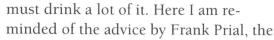

must drink a lot of it. Here I am reminded of the advice by Frank Prial, the wine editor for *The New York Times*—"Just bear in mind the old adage: There is no substitute for opening bottles" (p. 103).

Of course, if connoisseurship came purely from experience, all medical teachers already would be connoisseurs of teaching given the hundreds of hours they spend each year in **lectures**, **group discussions**, **morning report**, **teaching rounds**, and teaching at the **bedside**. The catch is that one must see as well as look! An educational connoisseur can see what is subtle, complex, and important in the **teaching–learning process**, and this requires knowledge about it. The word "connoisseur" is derived from the Latin, *cognoscere*, "to get acquainted with or to know thoroughly." Thus, connoisseur shares the same root as the word "cognition." The need to be knowledgeable was highlighted by the antiques editor for *The New York Times*, Rita Reif, who wrote that Charles Santore, a connoisseur of Windsor chairs, "relies upon his own educated eye, a great deal of acquired knowledge, and common sense to identify the Windsor designs he encounters" (p. 36).

The benefit of becoming a connoisseur of teaching is that you can learn about teaching in every educational encounter, whether you are the teacher, the learner, or an observer. As an educational connoisseur, you will be able to see what works and does not work. What helps students learn? What interferes with learning? In other words, you will be able to generate your own data base. This is helpful because one's own facts are much more powerful instruments of change than are facts generated and presented by an outside expert.

In *147 Practical Tips for Teaching Professors* Magnan (1989) suggests that teachers should observe each other teach, taking notes and sitting down together to discuss what occurred. When possible, two colleagues should observe a third teacher in action. Then all three could discuss their approaches to teaching the same material.

Be aware that there are risks in becoming a connoisseur. You will develop less tolerance for mediocre teaching; on the other hand, you will be highly appreciative when good teaching produces high levels of learning. Also, be cautious in judging the teaching you observe. Benjamin DeMott, a well–known professor of English, was asked to evaluate a seminar and wrote in his notes that the leader and one participant dominated the discussion. It was not until near the end of the session that others became involved. After class, DeMott admitted how badly he had misjudged the group at first, and the leader explained:

> I'm afraid it was your fault, sort of. It's a wonderful group, everybody extremely close. Lots of trust. We talked about your coming and—frankly—they hated it. Wrecking the chemistry and breaking down what they'd built up. I knew we were going to be stiff, it was just a question of when it would stop.

DeMott drew a good–sized X through his evaluation notes and wrote beneath it a message to himself: YOU DON'T KNOW A THING (p. 62).

CONTINUING MEDICAL EDUCATION

CME is a wimp activity! By this, I mean that little is expected—by the teacher or the learner. Much of it is offered in resort settings with a schedule to highlight the recreational activities. In my state, Utah, winter courses may meet early morning and early evening so that participants can ski all day. Also, teachers rarely challenge the learners. The dominant **method** of **teaching** is the "I talk—You listen" **lecture** with little learner participation. Much of the time, the **slides** are on and the lights are off—a condition not conducive to learning.

My theory is that physicians are exposed to an over-abundance of **stress** in medical school and residency training. Now that they are in practice, which has its own set of stresses, they want low stress education. However, *optimal stress* that challenges without threatening would produce more learning.

Drug companies also contribute to less–than–optimal learning. One pharmaceutical company paid a medical school to prepare and accredit a monograph on antihistamines. That monograph was distributed to physicians with a package of material promoting their new drug and with forms for them to request CME credit from the medical school after prescribing the drug and reporting on the results (Wilkes and Shuchman 1989). I question whether participating physicians felt motivated to put in the effort necessary to learn.

It is not my goal to change these practices. Change will occur only when medical schools and residencies produce truly lifelong learners who have not been turned off by their medical education. But I would like to see one small change in CME programs. I would like to see the typical "happiness" survey (see **teacher evaluation**) add the following items:

1.   What, if anything, did the instructor intend for you to do differently or better?

2.   Do you plan to do it?

3.   Why or why not?

If instructors were shown this evaluation format in advance of the presentation, they could see the emphasis on the learner's performance rather than on their own. Regardless of the evaluation format, a question all CME teachers should ask themselves is, "What impact do I want to have on the participants?"

THE CONVERSATION OF MEDICINE

To teach is to create a space in which the community of truth is practiced (Palmer 1990, p.12).

Dr. Lewis Thomas observed that science is taught as if its facts were somehow superior to the facts in other scholarly disciplines, even though every field of science is incomplete (1982). The same is true of medicine. The uncertainties of medicine were highlighted by Bursztajn *et al.* who described a "probabilistic paradigm" in their thoughtful book, *Medical Choice, Medical Chances* (1981). Medical teachers should consider that there may not be a universal structure behind "knowledge," but rather a temporary consensus arrived at by the medical community. If we are really concerned with training physicians for the twenty–first century, medical schools will be most effective when their students actively participate in the continuous conversation that occurs in medicine (Bruffee 1984).

There is a **myth of medical education** that students

have to learn the vocabulary of medicine before they begin to participate in its discussion. It is of course important that medical students learn a vocabulary, but they need not memorize a dictionary (Bishop 1984)! *This vocabulary can be learned in the process of medical problem solving.* As described by one faculty developer,

> Good teaching will help more and more people learn to speak and listen in the community of truth, to understand that truth is not in the conclusions so much as in the process of conversation itself, that if you want to be "in truth" you must be in the conversation (Palmer 1990, p. 12).

One **metaphor** I find helpful is to compare a school to a cocktail party. A newcomer enters a room where various conversations are occurring in clusters. When the newcomer walks up to a small group, he first must listen to find out what the conversation is about. Soon, he feels ready to contribute to the dialogue. At some point, a few people leave the group for another and others arrive. Eventually, our "newcomer" leaves the group to join another cluster. The medical school is one giant cocktail party where the conversation of medicine occurs in various courses and clinical rotations. This same conversation also goes on elsewhere, wherever medicine is practiced. Perhaps this is why Dr. Lloyd Smith warned us that one of the dangers of current medical education is that it leads to graduation from medical school. In his view, "The true physician never graduates from medical school; he simply transfers" (Smith 1985).

COOK'S LEARNING THEORIES

In a clever editorial, Richard I. Cook, who teaches in the Department of Anesthesiology at the Ohio State

University, described five medical lecture styles, each based on learning theories unrecognized by educational theorists. My department chairman sent me a copy of this article because she noticed that Cook referenced *The Physician as Teacher,* co–written with Thomas L. Schwenk, to support his notion that medical teachers' lecture styles are derived from their personal experiences as students and teachers, and may have no basis in educational theory. These are Cook's five medical lecture styles:

1. The *Passive Diffusion Theory* supposes that the lecture is a process akin to a passive diffusion across a semi-permeable membrane: there is a paucity of knowledge on the medical student's side, a surfeit of knowledge on the medical teacher's side, and a membrane between them. The purpose of a lecture is to provide a high gradient of knowledge to cause diffusion, thus increasing concentration on the student's side. Medical lecturers who adhere to this theory put much emphasis on the concentration of medical information to make the gradient as high as possible.

2. The *Receptor Theory* is based on the recognition that medical students have highly selective knowledge receptors and the role of the teacher is to package course materials to match the receptor affinity. These lecturers place a greater emphasis on format than do diffusionists.

3. The *Queueing Theory* postulates that students have a limited memory, consisting of slots that contain data items. Some teachers who subscribe to this theory believe in the last in–first out (LIFO) model and others the first in–first out (FIFO) model. LIFO lectures prefer to teach immediately before an examination and FIFO lecturers prefer to teach at the beginning of the academic term.

4.   The *Vigilance Theory* recognizes the need to get the students' attention with pop quizzes and horror stories about missed diagnoses. By frightening students, you can keep students on their toes.

5.   *Nihilism* is not considered by some to be a theory. Nihilists do not believe that lectures can produce learning. Although lectures may be unproductive, they still are necessary to maintain medical tradition. B.F. Skinner referred to the lecture as "**platform chicanery**."

Cook suggests that lecture style reveals a teacher's underlying theory of medical student learning and that "if the majority of medical lecturers remain untrained in education in general and lecturing in particular, new (but not necessarily effective) styles will evolve." While I welcome Cook's inference that training in education could be helpful to medical teachers, I feel obliged to refer to chapter one of *The Physician as Teacher*, in which Dr. Schwenk and I admit that many well–intentioned efforts at developing the teaching skills of physicians have been less than successful because faculty are asked to accept educational principles that are too theoretical. Medical education needs learning theories and educational principles adapted for the realities of the medical information explosion and the demands to train physicians for the twenty–first century.

CRITICISM OF MEDICAL EDUCATION

Dr. Lawrence K. Altman, the science editor for *The New York Times*, reviewed a number of complaints from prominent medical educators about medical education. One target is the **lecture**. For example, David E. Rogers, the former dean of the Johns Hopkins Medical School, reported that students were being lectured to death. Fred T.

Valentine, an infectious disease specialist at New York University, recommended that teachers put less emphasis on facts and more emphasis on correlating information when they lecture so that students will understand the subject: "...the better one understands a subject the less he has to memorize" (1982, p. 21).

Another target is the failure of medical schools to foster humanism in medicine. Lewis Thomas, chancellor of the Memorial–Sloan Kettering Cancer Center, accused medical school admission committees of playing a major role in the de–emphasis of the humanities in premedical education. Daniel C. Tosteson, dean of the Harvard Medical School, introduced the "new pathway" **problem–based, student–centered** curriculum with hopes of putting more emphasis on the need for compassion and understanding in treating patients.

Many other members of the medical education establishment have criticized medical education and have focused on the two issues of information overload and humanism in medicine. Those especially worth listening to include:

1.   Ludwig W. **Eichna** completed four years of medical school after retiring as the Chairman of Medicine at the State University of New York, Downstate Medical Center. One of his main complaints was the emphasis on accumulating facts: "Fact is king.... The gobs of facts delivered during the (first two) years leave little time for thinking" (1980, p. 729). A symptom of this problem is the "student syndicate" that arranges for a tape recorder in the front row so that lectures can be transcribed, typed, and sold to students, who stay home to study the transcripts!

     Eichna recognizes that facts are essential because problems cannot be solved without the sequential arrangement of facts. But, the concept of learning facts to pass examinations must be replaced with the concept of learning facts to solve problems.

2. Jerome P. Kassirer of the Tufts–New England Medical Center complains that clinical teachers do not preach what they practice! What they practice—which works—is the forming of diagnostic hypotheses based on minimal findings that are used to gather additional relevant data. By an "iterative process," hypotheses are confirmed or eliminated, and those that remain are made progressively more specific. What they preach is different:

> Instead, students are expected to learn diagnostic **problem solving** by reading textbooks, studying clinical pathological conferences, attending conferences dominated by case presentations, or observing physicians at work and rediscovering the process of clinical reasoning by trial and error (1983, p. 921).

Kassirer suggests that clinical teachers preach what they practice. Let a student present only a patient's age, sex, race, and reason for seeking medical attention and instruct the team members to ask questions that will produce more data. But students who ask for data should be prepared to explain why they asked the question and what they expect to learn from it. After getting information, they should be prepared to explain what they learned and whether it changed their thinking. Since patients do not "present their case" to their doctors, this iterative approach simulates actual medical practice and provides students with the opportunity to develop data collection strategies (see **simulation**).

3.   George L. Engel, a professor of Psychiatry and Medicine at the University of Rochester, has visited some seventy medical schools in the United States and Canada since 1970. He found that few students are observed and critiqued interviewing a patient during their junior or senior years. In addition, few of them observe an experienced clinician conduct a first–contact patient interview. Engel asks, "What if music students were taught to play their instruments as medical students are taught to interview?"

> If musicians learned to play their instruments as physicians learn to interview patients, the procedure would consist of presenting in lectures or maybe in a demonstration or two the theory and mechanisms of the music–producing ability of the instrument and telling him to produce a melody. The instructor, of course, would not be present to observe or listen to the student's efforts but would be satisfied with the student's subsequent verbal report of what came out of the instrument (1982, p.12).

Engel complains that such an approach corresponds with the widespread practice in medical schools of sending a student to "get the history" from a patient and then to "report the 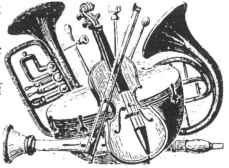 history" to the instructor. He strongly recommends that clinical instructors both demonstrate how to interview patients and observe student interviews so that they can provide **feedback**. Unfortunately, in many medical schools, this type of instruction may occur only in the preclinical years and is not repeated in the clinical years when the students are actually interviewing real patients.

4. Eugene W. Linfors and Francis A. Neelson of the Duke Medical Center telephoned chief medical residents in fourteen medical centers and found that only five percent estimated that the majority of their case presentations occurred in the presence of the patient. Based on their experiences and those reported in other studies, it appears that, "There has been a pervasive translocation of teaching activity away from the bedside and into the classroom" (1980, p. 1231). They recommend a return to **bedside teaching** for four reasons:

> "The patient can be seen as an individual."

> "The teaching function of the doctor can be demonstrated."

> "Contact with the patient is prolonged."

> "The human dimension can be incorporated into the clinical learning process."

I believe the criticisms of these medical educators are constructive. If students are encouraged by their teachers to look at medical facts as a means rather than an end, and if they are expected to gather patient facts in the iterative approach, then they will become the continuous learners that physicians of the twenty–first century are expected to be. If teachers demonstrate and observe patient interactions and conduct more teaching at the bedside, then our students can become the kind of caring physicians needed to handle the human dimensions in an increasingly technological system of care.

DEMONSTRATING

One creative **technique** that can be used to attract attention at the start of a lecture or to maintain **attention** as minds begin to wander in the middle of a presentation is to use a demonstration. This technique of teaching includes examples, experiments, or some actual performance to illustrate a principle or to show how to do something. Its advantages include bridging the gap between theory and practice, preparing students to do the same activity, and providing a memorable experience.

I strongly recommend that teachers test all the equipment in advance and practice as often as necessary so that the demonstration is conducted smoothly. Before the demonstration, explain what to look for. Review the major points at the end of the demonstration. These principles of good teaching were modeled by a master chef during a cooking class:

> Giving the whys at every step is the mark of a good teacher. 'Can you believe I've taken this long to spread this cake batter?' Flo Braker, the author of *The Simple Art of Perfect Baking*, asked at a recent demonstration, after compressing a whole chapter into the explanation of one recipe. Braker was so eager for students to understand what she was saying that she carried around bowls of batter and meringue to show exactly the consistency she recommended. 'To make a meringue mount fully, wipe the bowl with a few drops of white vinegar and don't start adding the sugar until the egg whites begin to foam.' She refused to move on to the next step until she was sure everyone was following her. I've been to demonstrations where I didn't know what

was going on and was too embarrassed to ask. Braker encouraged stupid questions (Kummer 1985, p. 98).

Please remember that the only stupid questions are those not asked—or answered.

DOCTOR FOX

The validity of the **lecture** was questioned by B. F. Skinner in *Walden Two*. In that futuristic novel, a member of a utopian community tells a visitor that the lecture became obsolete with the invention of printing: "Why don't you just hand printed lectures to your students? Yes, I know. Because they won't read them. A fine institution it is that must solve that problem with platform chicanery." Is lecturing **platform chicanery**? In a study of the effect of the instructor's personality on student ratings, a professional actor was programmed to teach charismatically, but without substance, on a topic about which he knew nothing: "Mathematical Game Theory as Applied to Physician Education."

The actor, introduced to the unsuspecting audience as Dr. Myron L. Fox, was trained by the investigators to say nothing, but to say it beautifully. Almost all the physicians (who viewed the live lecture) and the students in a graduate school of education (who viewed its videotape) gave Dr. Fox high ratings as a teacher. Specifically, they thought he used good examples, was well–organized, and stimulated their thinking. No one detected the lecture for the charade that it was, and one person even claimed familiarity with the speaker's publications (Naftulin, Ware, and Donnelly).

In a follow-up study, Ware and Williams admitted that the original Dr. Fox study went too far in claiming that participants had been seduced into thinking they had learned. They pointed out that the subjects had not been asked to rate their learning gains and no measure of learning was used. So, the same actor was hired to lecture to medical students on the biochemistry of learning, and the students were tested on the material without warning two weeks later. The students were randomly assigned to six groups: Dr. Fox delivered a high–content lecture (26 facts), a medium–content lecture (14 facts), and low–content lecture (4 facts), and each level of content was presented with a high–seduction or low–seduction teaching style. High seduction teaching behaviors included enthusiasm, humor, friendliness, and expressiveness. Low seduction was monotonous and boring (see **boring teachers**).

In general, students who viewed high seduction lectures performed better than did students who viewed low seduction lectures, and students who viewed high–content lectures did better than students who viewed low–content lectures. What intrigued me was that the low–content, high seduction group equalled the high–content, low seduction group on the test. The test consisted of the 26 items presented in the high–content lecture. The low–content group had received only four of those facts, yet the performance of both groups was the same.

Numerous Dr. Fox studies have since been conducted. In a synthesis of these studies, Abrami and colleagues found that, overall, the instructor's expressiveness had a substantial impact on student ratings. Also, the amount of content had substantial impact on student learning, but no conclusive impact on ratings. Since being expressive at least does not lower student test results and teaching an optimal level on content does not lower student ratings of the instructor, why not do both? In a variation of the Dr. Fox effect, the Department of Physiology at the University of Utah School of Medicine challenged me to give one of their lectures. See **physiology chicken coop** to discover what happened!

DOUBLE O SEVENS

The need for reliable and valid student evaluation was highlighted by Dr. Perri Klass (1985) in a story about a emergency room patient with lower back pain. When asked by an attending physician, "So, what's your diagnosis?" a medical student says without hesitation, "Ruptured aortic aneurysm." "That's right!" says the attending. "How on earth did you figure it out?" The student responds, "So what else gives you low back pain?"

This medical student may become a "007 doctor," licensed to kill…unless his teachers carefully evaluate his competence. The problem is that, because students do not want negative evaluations, they may play the **pretend to know game**, sabotaging your efforts to assess their fund of knowledge. Also, as pointed out by Dr. George Engel (1982), if you rely upon self–report to evaluate clinical skills, students may not volunteer their deficiencies. To ensure that we are not graduating doctors licensed to kill, we must directly observe their clinical skills.

According to a study sponsored by the Clinical Evaluation Project of the Association of American Medical Colleges (1983), although faculty are able to reliably identify failing students, they do not handle them well. In other words, they know who the 007s are, but do not know what to do with them. What needs to be done is to document the student's weaknesses, to make explicit requirements for satisfactory performance, and to specify the criteria by which judgments will be made (see **feedback, giving**). If the student's subsequent performance does not meet the criteria, the faculty must consider the student's dismissal.

Faculty should not fear legal action if they follow their own written policies and procedures, including providing fair opportunities for appeal. What they *should* fear is sending a 007 to a residency program, hoping that the faculty there will protect the public. If we are to provide good physicians for the twenty–first century, then **student evaluation** must be an integral part of the educational process. Proper evaluation of medical students is important not only to them and their teachers, but also to graduate medical education programs that will accept them as residents.

As an example of helpful evaluation, the University of Illinois College of Medicine reported that students rarely fail the second–year physical diagnosis course in which they examine a patient under the supervision of a physician teacher. However, one student's performance was so poor that his teacher refused to pass him. The student's questions on the history were too detailed, he allowed the patient to ramble, and he omitted key questions. The physical examination was awkward, unsystematic, and full of omissions. The student was given specific feedback and a week of intensive practice before re–testing. On the re–test, his performance was not just satisfactory but, in fact, was very good (Whalen 1985).

Later, when this student was on his first clinical rotation, he called the teacher who had failed him to say thank you. The point here is that we do no favors to marginal students by passing them. Even students understand that!

EICHNA

In September 1975, the State University of New York, Downstate Medical Center, enrolled an unusual freshman medical student. Ludwig W. Eichna, after retiring from the chairmanship of the Department of Medicine, decided to return to medical school. He passed all the courses and graduated in May 1979. Subsequently, he published in *The New England Journal of Medicine* his observations as a student (1980) and his views concerning a medical curriculum for the 1980s (1981).

Why would a seasoned scholar, clinician, and teacher subject himself to take everything that the regular students went through, including:

> lectures, conferences, seminars, reports, laboratories, patient work–ups and presentations, operating–room and delivery–room duties, nights and weekends on call, and all examinations, written and oral, including National Board Examinations Parts I and II (1980, p. 727)?

Eichna explained that he had felt increasingly dissatisfied with the courses and results of medical education and wanted to experience first hand where the problems lay. Based on his personal experience, he developed eight principles that should, but in his opinion currently do not, guide a medical school education:

1. *The focus and first priority of medical education is the patient.* In practice, he found that too often the patient is a secondary consideration. Faculty distort this principle by letting personal interests take over, with each faculty member insisting that his specialty receive favored treatment.

2. *The profession of medicine is a science, humanely conducted.* Yet, he found that from the first day of medical school, students are given the message that the sciences are secondary to the real thing, a chore to be endured before patient contact.

3. *Learning is a thinking, **problem solving** process that requires time.* Eichna claims that medical education today involves too little thinking and problem solving. The curriculum packs too many facts in too little time. Here he finds that the faculty are not solely at fault; students arrive with the habit of memorizing facts for the examination.

4. *Medical education is a continuum, binding college education, medical–school education, and postgraduate house–officership training into a unified whole.* However, from his perspective, each phase of education goes its own way with little or no coordination.

5. *Learning medicine requires a proper balance between **apprenticeship** (practical) training and formal teaching in lectures and seminars.* This balance does not now exist. Eichna is not in favor of abolishing all **lectures**—only bad ones! He also observes that rounds downgrade clinical skill in favor of laboratory numbers.

6. *Education requires evaluation procedures that correctly assess progress and competence.* Yet, he did not see fellow students properly tested in biomedical science, clinical knowledge, clinical skills and problem solving. In practice, **student tests** assessed memorization of facts.

7. *Medical school education requires adherence to a standard of excellence.* Eichna thought he saw a lowering of academic standards, typified by the "pass–fail"

system and by lowering the passing grade. In effect, poorer students who pull down the mean are setting standards.

8.   *The profession of medicine demands at all levels, specifically including that of medical students, the highest ethical conduct.* Here was Eichna's greatest indictment: "I have saved this principle until last because of its importance and the almost total neglect of it in medical–school education" (p. 733). It was the lack of medical ethics as a subject to be taught by daily practice that most offended Dr. Eichna.

Well, what do you think? To be honest, if I did not know that Dr. Eichna had returned to medical school, I would have thought that this retired Chairman of Medicine was an old crank! Even knowing that he had repeated four years of medical school, I still might have dismissed him. But, hearing him speak at the Generalists in Medical Education meeting in 1982 made me realize what a caring, concerned person he is. It is hard to ignore his warning that, "these deficiencies and faults exist at all medical schools. They are there, and they cry for correction" (p. 734).

Since Dr. Eichna pronounced the patient as morbid, what treatment did he prescribe? He suggests recognizing that the curriculum is for the students, not for the faculty: the biological–science faculty should stop underestimating medical students and spoon feeding them and the clinical faculty should stop overestimating students and allowing them to participate in clinical care before they are ready. When students are ready for clinical responsibility, the curriculum should emphasize problem solving, patient care skills, and medical ethics. Looking at his year–by–year model curriculum, it seems to me that the aforementioned eight principles which should guide medical education would be operational if faculty adhered to the **teaching–learning**

process advocated in this book, a viewpoint which recognizes that if the learner didn't learn, then the teacher didn't teach.

ENTHUSIASM

In *The Log from the Sea of Cortez*, John Steinbeck reflected on the role of enthusiasm in science while collecting marine animals during low tide:

> At first the rocks are bright and every living animal makes his mark on attention. The picture is wide and colored and beautiful. But after an hour and a half the attention centers weary, the colors fade, and the field is likely to narrow to an individual animal. Here one may observe his own world narrowed down until interest and, with it, observation flicker and go out. And what if with age this weariness become permanent and observation dim out and not recover? Can this be what happens to so many men of science? Enthusiasm, interest, sharpness, dulled with weariness until finally they retire into easy didacticism?... We have known so many professors who once carried their listeners high on their single enthusiasm, and have seen these same men finally settle back comfortably into lectures prepared years before and never vary them again.

In teaching, as in science, enthusiasm is a key ingredient for success. In a review of **clinical teaching**, Irby (1978) identified enthusiasm as one of seven important factors (the others were organization and clarity of presentation, instructor knowledge, group instructional skills, clinical supervision skills, clinical competence, and **role modeling**). In his own study of 320 medical students evaluating 230 faculty members and residents in Obstetrics and Gynecology, Irby found four teaching behaviors that correlated most strongly with overall teaching effectiveness (1981):

1.   Is enthusiastic and stimulating.

2.   Establishes rapport.

3.   Actively involves students.

4.   Provides direction and **feedback**.

FACULTY DEVELOPMENT PROBLEMS

If you think the cost of education is high, think about ignorance (Derek Bok, President, Harvard University).

There are several problems that obstruct efforts to help medical faculty become better teachers. First, low extrinsic rewards may de–motivate faculty to make any effort to improve their teaching. In a survey of faculty in my medical school, I was not surprised to discover that no one believes improved teaching will lead to higher salary. But, I was surprised by how few faculty believe that a fair portion of their salary corresponds to the time they take to teach, including preparation time. With regard to intrinsic rewards, they were not sure whether good teachers are recognized and held in high esteem in the medical school and were not sure whether good teaching was appreciated by their superiors. Without such intrinsic rewards, it can be difficult to motivate faculty to improve their teaching (see **faculty development strategies**).

Another obstacle to faculty development of teaching skills is faculty skepticism that teaching can be improved. If good teachers are born, not made, then trying to improve teaching could be a waste of time (see **myths of teaching**). Many faculty may also believe that they already know all there is to know about teaching. Given the number of years medical teachers have spent in the educational system (at least twenty years as a learner!), this "know it all" attitude is understandable. Even when faculty think teaching is a skill that can be learned, they may not think that "faculty developers" are credible resources. When the faculty

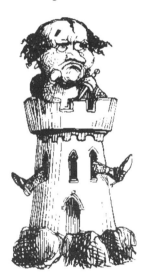

developer is an M.D. who has chosen medical education as his "specialty," medical colleagues often find that choice suspicious. When the faculty developer is a Ph.D. in education, medical faculty can doubt this person's ability to understand science and medicine.

How warranted is this credibility gap? Most faculty developers have much to offer. But, some M.D. faculty developers have axes to grind and cannot go beyond their personal experiences and prejudices about medical education. Also, some Ph.D. educators do not relate what they learned in graduate schools of education to the medical school setting. For these reasons, M.D. and Ph.D. faculty developers must observe medical teaching in action. They should attend medical lectures and grand rounds, observe continuing medical education programs, follow ward teams on hospital rounds, stand in the operating room, and visit the offices of preceptors.

This raises one more problem. Many medical teachers do not like to be seen in action. In other words, teaching is a personal activity and being watched can be discomforting, understandably so. But, if I do not observe it, on what basis can I recommend improvement?

FACULTY DEVELOPMENT STRATEGIES

There are five approaches to the development of medical school **teaching** skills:

1.   Through a system of *rewards*, faculty will improve their own teaching because it is worth their while. Faculty developers should recognize that there are two kinds of rewards: extrinsic and intrinsic. Extrinsic rewards, such as money, are important because their absence is de–motivating. If faculty do not feel they are paid to teach and that better teaching can lead to advancement and promotion, then they will not be motivated to teach more effectively. Intrinsic rewards are important because a sense of ownership in the institution and a feeling of pride in its teaching program will motivate faculty to improve their teaching skills. Unfortunately, some medical school administrators think that the "teacher of the year" award is an intrinsic reward. However, this is like offering a "Druid of the Year" award in the Mojave Desert. If you want Druids, you must grow forests (Eble 1984).

2.   If they receive *assistance*, faculty can learn how to improve their teaching skills. For this strategy to work, faculty must perceive that educational assistance is available and credible. However, educational consultants often are located in an "Office of Medical Education Research," where educational research rather than educational service may be the top priority. For an excellent guide to planning

faculty development workshops, refer to Bland (1980). Also, see **teacher training**.

3. *Feedback* on their teaching strengths and weaknesses can help faculty make the necessary adjustments to improve their teaching. We know that feedback (see **feedback, getting** and **feedback, giving**) is more useful when it is timely. Do course teachers see their **student ratings** in the middle of the next academic period? Do clinical teachers see their evaluations two or three months after the rotation? An even more critical question is, do faculty value student ratings? And, is there a comprehensive system of **teacher evaluation** that makes use of colleague and self–assessment?

4. Faculty can learn how to teach more effectively by developing a taste for teaching, a process known as *educational connoisseurship*. By paying attention to the **teaching–learning process**, faculty can learn about the subject of teaching every time a medical subject is being taught. The next time you are bored or stimulated by Grand Rounds, ask yourself, "What is going on here and what does this tell me about my own teaching practices?" (see **connoisseurship**)

5. Teaching will improve if faculty feel free to become *creative*, trying to be both useful in what they teach and novel in how they teach. Medical schools do not tolerate charlatans, who are novel, but not useful; however, pedantic bores, who are useful, but not novel, are quite acceptable. Although the promotion policy will typically state that faculty members must excel in either research, service, or teaching and perform satisfactorily in the other two areas, in reality, promotion reviews often pay lip service to teaching and focus primarily on research.

I have developed a survey to measure the degree to which faculty think these strategies are used in their institutions. As one might expect, typical responses indicate that the rewards strategy is used least to promote faculty development of teaching skills. Connoisseurship and creativity are rated the highest, with faculty perceiving that they learn from teaching experience and try to be innovative in their approaches to teaching. Depending upon the educational support available in a department or school–at–large and the system of evaluating teaching, assistance and feedback scores vary greatly.

I think it is realistic for department chairmen to promote faculty development of teaching skills by…

1.   taking teaching into consideration when considering faculty promotion;

2.   on a regular basis, sponsoring a workshop on teaching skills;

3.   observing teaching and giving faculty feedback;

4.   asking faculty to assess and discuss colleague performance; and

5   tolerating neither pedantic bores nor charlatans.

FAILURE OF THE THREE MINUTE LECTURE

The "three minute lecture" is a **method** of teaching frequently used by physicians during **teaching rounds** with the aim of imparting information. While consulting to the University of Missouri–Kansas City, Department of Family Medicine, I challenged one of their faculty, Dr. Len Scarpinato, who gave a three minute lecture during rounds, to test the efficacy of this method. During rounds, Dr.

Scarpinato had lectured on the potential deleterious implications of four drugs being used in a diabetic renal insufficiency patient and commented on two other agents.

Without warning, the students and residents present in rounds the next morning were handed slips of paper and asked to recall the names of the drugs, the specific comment made on each, and the comments made about two other agents (maximum score = 10). Thirteen students and residents responded, with a range of 0–8. The mean was 5 and the median 6. The low retention rate caused Dr. Scarpinato to sharply curtail the use of three minute lectures during teaching rounds (Scarpinato and Whitman 1990).

While I am not opposed to giving information during rounds, I am in favor of limiting the amount of information given. By adapting **information giving** tips that work with patients, we can increase the probability that what is transmitted will be received.

FEEDBACK TO CLINICAL TEACHERS

Student rating forms are the most popular format of giving faculty feedback on their teaching. However, clinical teachers typically do not find these useful. Medical faculty at the University of Toronto conducted a study to determine the effectiveness of a group discussion format for faculty feedback. In this approach, a skilled group leader guided discussions with small groups of students, resulting in a summary report submitted to the teacher (Tiberius *et al.* 1989). In their investigation, the influence of feedback was studied over four clinical rotations, each of two month's duration. They compared the effect of ratings alone shared with faculty, ratings alone not given to faculty, and ratings plus group discussion.

They found that feedback from student ratings alone had no sustained effect on teaching, as indicated by subsequent student ratings. However, student feedback may have had some beneficial effect because the student ratings of faculty who received no feedback decreased over time! On the other hand, the combination of student ratings and the group discussion format led to improved student ratings, improvement characterized by the investigators as "dramatic *and* sustained over successive groups of students" (p. 676).

An important conclusion of their study is that feedback to faculty can enhance the collaborative relationship, especially if the feedback lets teachers know what students think and feel and lets students know that someone is listening. Tiberius and colleagues recommend that clinical faculty and medical students participate (p. 679) "in a *real* conversation, in which feedback proceeded in both directions..." (see **the conversation of medicine**).

Real conversation was promoted by faculty in the Department of Family Medicine at the State University of New York at Buffalo who developed a creative approach to giving feedback to their clinical preceptors in private practice. Four groups of twelve second–year students each were questioned in a videotaped session. Issues addressed included their expectations and experiences during biweekly placement in a physician's office. Editing produced a twenty–minute videotape that was shown at a Sunday brunch meeting of preceptors, providing an opportunity to communicate student feedback in a non–threatening fashion (Lenkei and Bissonette 1989).

FEEDBACK, GETTING

Using feedback to improve clinical practice is a skill that should be learned during medical school and residency

training. Some clinical teachers are **sharks**, and getting
feedback from them can be dangerous. I tell medical students
and residents that if they do not develop the skill of using
feedback, they may find themselves embattled throughout
their medical career. My point is that, even when feedback is
not given artfully, it still can be useful. As Ben Franklin once
said, "Things which hurt, instruct." Nevertheless, I am
willing to acknowledge that sometimes it is difficult to make
use of feedback. Here I am reminded of Mark Twain's criticism of James Fenimore Cooper: "In one place in Deerslayer,
and in the restricted space of two–thirds of a page, Cooper
has scored 114 offences against literary art out of a possible
115. It breaks the record." It is doubtful that Cooper would
have found this feedback helpful.

It probably would be easier to make use of negative
feedback if the same person occasionally gave us positive
feedback. However, people getting feedback should realize
that some teachers only give negative feedback. Good performance is expected and taken for granted. This pattern starts
early in life. For a moment, think your
way back to the first grade.
The class is divided into
three reading groups:
bluebirds, robins, and
vultures. You, of course,
are in the bluebird
group, and the reading
teacher is calling on
bluebirds to read out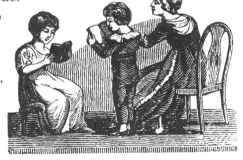
loud. You are waiting for your turn, feeling anxious because
you want to do well. When your turn comes, you take a deep
breath and read beautifully—no errors, good pronunciation,
and so on. You stop, feeling relief at doing a good job, and
hear the teacher say… "Next."

Clinicians in training and in practice should be aware that some feedback will be off target. The person giving it is wrong! Of course, the whole world cannot always be wrong, and some of the negative feedback, hurtful as it is, will be valid. In recognition of these differences, I find helpful the words of the Amherst poet, Robert Francis, a contemporary of Robert Frost. Although Francis is well–regarded today, he had years of literary rejection. Frost's success and popularity must have galled him. While he accepted some of the criticism as accurate, he might have stopped writing had he agreed with all of it. The following words appeared in his journal on March 17, 1932:

> Years ago I read of a highly skilled craftsman who was employed to remove excessive coatings of varnish from old paintings. He did the rubbing away with his thumb, a thumb that had grown extraordinarily sensitive to distinguish the feeling of varnish from the feeling of paint, and which had also grown, naturally, though paradoxically, callous. That callous, sensitive thumb has been to me a symbol of the well–adapted artist in his reaction to criticism—or to all life, for that matter.

FEEDBACK, GIVING

One of the most impactful **teaching** behaviors in clinical education is to give medical students or residents feedback on their performance. By feedback, I mean information about current performance that can be used to improve it in the future. "Current" performance is subjective, but in a clinical setting I think that an episode more than forty–eight hours old is ancient history—at least from the viewpoint of the medical student or resident. When giving feedback, clinical instructors should consider meaningful positive as well as negative performance. What did the learner do right that you want him to do again? What did he do wrong that needs to be changed? This does not mean that you should always "tell it like it is." Tell it like it is when "it" is worth mentioning. On the other hand, avoid "telling it like it isn't." Some teachers downplay the negative because they want to be liked by students and residents, and others downplay the positive because they want to keep students and residents on their toes.

When giving positive or negative feedback, it is almost always helpful to begin with the learner. Ask for his assessment. This provides you with an opportunity to find out how insightful the learner is, and it enables learners to develop criteria. Becoming insightful about one's own performance and developing the ability to self–assess performance is critical to producing the lifelong learners we want practicing in the twenty–first century. Because people may do the wrong thing for good reasons or the right thing for the wrong reasons, beginning with the learner helps you assess their performance more accurately (see **double o sevens**).

Timing is critical to effective feedback. In general, feedback should be given as soon after the event as possible. However, this strategy is not always possible or even desirable. Some feedback, particularly negative, might be better handled in private. Also, both parties need sufficient time. If you or the resident have a foot out the door, then this is not a good time. Or, if either person is very upset—often the case when negative feedback is warranted—then it might be better to put off the feedback until emotions are under control. Should you choose to delay feedback for any reason, let the person know that there will be feedback soon, perhaps later that day or the next morning.

Most medical students and residents will be grateful for your feedback. Others may be defensive...understandably so. In an ego–intensive environment, people are used to top performance. The best way to head off defensiveness is to "catch people doing something right" (Blanchard and Johnson 1982) as soon as possible so that you can give deserved positive feedback. When, and if, you want to give negative feedback, this will not be their first feedback from you. Most students and residents can take negative feedback if they perceive you as fair, *i.e.*, you call 'em the way you see 'em. They do not know this is the case if the first feedback they get from you is negative.

I hope you will avoid collusion—teachers and learners tacitly agreeing to avoid feedback.

GPEP REPORT

In 1984 the Association of American Medical Colleges published the General Professional Education of the Physician (GPEP) Report. Many medical schools have discussed this report, and every medical teacher should become familiar with its six recommendations regarding the role of medical school faculty:

1. Medical school deans should identify and designate an interdisciplinary and interdepartmental organization of faculty members to formulate a coherent and comprehensive educational program for medical students and to select the instructional and evaluation methods to be used.

2. The educational program for medical students should have a defined budget that provides resources needed for its conduct.

3. Faculty members should have the time and opportunity to establish a **mentor** relationship with individual students.

4. Medical schools should establish programs to assist members of the faculty to expand their teaching capabilities. (see **teacher training**)

5. Medical faculties should provide support and guidance to enhance the personal development of each medical student.

6. Experience indicates that the commitment to education of deans and department chairmen greatly influences the behavior of faculty members in their institutions and their departments. (see **faculty development strategies**)

GROUP DISCUSSION

Without discussion, intellectual experience is only an exercise in a private gymnasium (Randolph Bourne).

The teacher's most significant role in a group discussion may be to teach students to teach themselves. Using the Socratic **metaphor**, Robert Segal says that the group discussion leader serves as a midwife to students pregnant with ideas. Thus, a good discussion leader does not directly convey what he knows, but uses what he knows to convey to students what they themselves already know or can learn (1979).

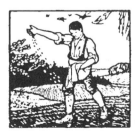 Of course, some group discussion leaders may feel more like a farmer than a midwife, sowing seeds that fall sometimes on fertile soil, sometimes on soil that is barren. Or, they may see themselves as Jehovah who breathes a soul into the clod!

According to Davis, Fry, and Alexander (1977), research on the discussion **method** suggests ten propositions:

1. The discussion method is conducive to eliciting higher levels of reflective thinking than is the **lecture** method.

2. The discussion method seems best for increasing **problem solving** and for dealing with **attitudinal change**.

3. When **student tests** only measure acquisition of facts, the lecture method and group discussions are equal.

4. When student tests are administered six months after course completion, information learned through discussion is retained better than the same information presented in lectures.

5. Able students profit more from group discussion than less able students.

6. Higher quality solutions result when discussions are led by a facilitative leader.

7. Students prefer group discussions over lectures when grades are not determined by multiple choice tests.

8. Group discussions are more effective than lectures in changing content–specific attitudes in directions desired by the teacher.

9. When students are assigned to argue for a point of view different from their own, their attitudes are apt to change.

10. The optimal size of a group discussion is between five and eight students.

HARVARD'S NEW PATHWAY

In 1985 the Harvard Medical School implemented an experimental curriculum to better prepare its graduates for practicing medicine in the twenty–first century (Harvard Medical School Office of Educational Development 1989). Instead of traditional lectures, the "New Pathway" uses **problem–based teaching** and **student–centered learning**. The main idea is for students in small groups to discuss patient cases designed to uncover what they do not know, but will have to know, to understand the problem. The teacher's role is to facilitate and guide the process during these tutorial sessions so that students can seek information on their own and teach each other (see **peer teaching**).

Since patient cases tend to cross disciplines, the first two years of the curriculum had to be organized along inter-disciplinary lines:

1.   *The Body* (histology, gross anatomy, radiology)

2.   *Metabolism of Matter and Energy* (biochemistry, physiology, pharmacology, and molecular biology)

3.   *Identity and Defense* (pathology, immunology, micro-biology, and infectious disease)

4.   *Life Cycle* (embryology and clinical genetics)

5.   *Information Processing and Behavior* (human brain and spinal cord, localization of function, neural transmission, autonomic nervous system)

6.   *Human Systems* (pathophysiology of organ systems)

7.   *The Patient and Doctor* (patient interviewing, medical sociology and anthropology, ethics, economics of health care delivery, epidemiology and biostatistics, decision analysis, critical reading of medical litera-ture, and health promotion and disease prevention)

This innovative curriculum, as well as the **New Mexico Experiment**, is an example of medical school reforms aimed at teaching medical students how to learn so that they will become lifelong learners.

HELPFUL CLINICAL TEACHERS

According to a survey of third and fourth year medical students, helpful clinical teachers do the following things (Stritter, Hain, and Grimes 1975):

1. Answer carefully and precisely questions raised by students. (see **questioning**)

2. Approach teaching with enthusiasm. (see **enthusiasm**)

3. Explain the basis for their actions and decisions. (see **problem solving**)

4. Provide students with opportunities to practice both technical and problem solving skills. (see **skills**)

5. Summarize major points. (see **remembering**)

6. Correct students when wrong without belittling. (see **feedback, giving**)

7. Demonstrate a genuine interest in students. (see **mentor**)

8. Strive to make difficult concepts easy to understand. (see **Raimi**)

9. Emphasize conceptual comprehension rather than merely factual recall. (see **knowledge**)

10. Willingly remain accessible to students. (see **professional intimacy**)

11. Provide competent patient care. (see **role model**)

12. Approach their teaching with dynamism and energy. (see **boring teachers**)

13. Prepare well for rounds and other contact with students. (see **morning report**)

14. Explain lucidly. (see **Kroenke's rules**)

15. Identify what they consider important. (see **useful**)

16. Discuss practical applications of knowledge and skills. (see **preceptor's agenda**)

HUMANISTIC BEHAVIOR

Can medical students and residents be taught to be humanistic? To test whether humanistic behavior could be enhanced, medical educators at the University of Connecticut demonstrated pre– and post–videotaped improvements by medical students and residents. While there is no guarantee that these physicians–in–training will later put these behaviors into practice, the results of this study give at least a ray of hope to future physicians (Sheehan 1989).

The primary teaching **technique** used in this program was the **role play** with individualized **feedback**. Each role play consisted of a scenario describing a medical–value conflict, and the medical students and residents were rotated through the roles of patient, physician, and observer. For example, in one scenario, a young man comes to a physician to have his marriage certificate signed. The physician knows that this person is sterile and that his fiancee would like to have children. He does not know whether this man has told his future bride. What should he say?

Humanistic behavior, like **attitudinal change**, is difficult to achieve. But, any possibility of achieving these **objectives** depends upon student involvement. Obviously, the **lecture** alone will not do it. The need to look for alternatives to the lecture method was highlighted by Dr. David E. Ness who used the discussion of short stories to teach about doctor–patient relationships (see **literature and medicine**).

INFORMATION GIVING

Physicians learn by experience how to give information to patients so that it is remembered. Because **clinical teaching is like clinical care**, they should consider adapting this experience to giving information to medical students and residents during **morning report** and **teaching rounds**. Specifically, clinical teachers should...

1. limit the amount of information given in any one session;

2. give the most important information first;

3. emphasize why the information is important;

4. check out if the information is understood;

5. use repetition for emphasis;

6. make instructions specific; and

7. provide options when possible.

INFORMATION OVERLOAD

Where is the wisdom we have lost in knowledge? Where is the knowledge we have lost in information? (T.S. Eliot).

Because medical knowledge is expanding and changing, information overload is a major problem in medical education. In the field of pharmacology, Riley (1984) highlighted the problem by comparing the indices of the 1980 and 1970 editions of Goodman and Gilman's *The*

Pharmacological Basis of Therapeutics. The 1980 edition dropped 300 drugs listed in the 1970 edition and added 800 new ones, for a net gain of 500 generic drugs.

Dr. Riley reviewed the 1981 course handouts and lecture notes at the Medical College of Georgia and identified 525 drug names, which would require learning 25 new drugs per week during the 20–week course. By analyzing commonly prescribed and prototypical drugs which appeared on course exams and the National Board of Medical Examinations, he developed the "200 drug list," which was reviewed and revised by a faculty committee. Subsequently, the pharmacology course focused on this list.

As a result of this change, learning responsibilities could be clearly defined at the start of this course, faculty reached consensus on what to teach, and there was no adverse effect on student performance on National Boards! The lesson for medical teachers in all disciplines is that, "Limiting the teaching material in this fashion (see **lecture paradox**) may actually enhance student learning and retention due to reduction in information overload" (Riley 1984, p. 511).

JOUBERT

(One) aspect of being a good physician comes from the term doctor, from the Latin docer, meaning teacher. A good physician has a lifelong commitment to learning, and teachers are lifelong students. Teaching is integral to all residency programs, reflecting that the best way to learn is by teaching (Miller 1990).

Joseph Joubert was born on May 7, 1754, the son of a French surgeon. He chose the profession of teaching and in 1809 was named Inspector General of Education, a post he held for six years. When he died in 1824, Joubert was considered one of France's great educator–philosophers. His supporter Chateaubriand, the Minister of Foreign Affairs, published Joubert's notebooks in 1838. The maxims and aphorisms sprinkled throughout his notebooks remain relevant today. Upon noticing Joubert's epigram "To teach is to learn twice" on a pamphlet on teaching published by the Mathematical Society of America, Ralph **Raimi**, a professor at the University of Rochester, wrote in *The New York Times,* "Quelle belle sentiment! Whatever sort of penseur Joubert may have been, he must have been a teacher too, for every teacher knows this: that we have never learned anything so well as when we have had to teach it."

"To teach is to learn twice" is a statement I repeat in workshops on teaching skills for residents when I want to impress upon them the fact that they will be the main beneficiaries of their own teaching. Here are some other Joubertisms to provoke your thinking about teaching:

- Are you listening to the ones who keep quiet?

- Big words claim too much attention.

- Yes, please cut up the pieces for me, but don't chew them.

- To know is to see inside oneself.

- Speak softly to be better heard by a deaf public.

- Everything has its poetry.

- The breath of the mind is attention.

KNOWLEDGE

Knowledge is one of three domains of **learning**, along with **attitudinal change** and **skills**. In a taxonomy of knowledge **objectives**, Bloom *et al.* identified six levels. The lowest level of knowledge objectives is learning *facts*. Anderson and Graham have estimated that medical students are expected to learn 50,000 facts during the first two years of medical school. Lloyd Smith, in his plenary presentation at the 1984 annual meeting of the Association of American Medical Colleges, commented that overdosing on facts is like giving thyroxine to a tadpole—one gets an instant frog, but unfortunately a rather small one.

The next level of knowledge objectives is *comprehension*, which expects more from a student than the ability to recite facts. Comprehension requires a learner to demonstrate understanding, explain information, and make generalizations. Sometimes, students already know the facts, and the teacher's aim is to help them comprehend their meaning. If a teacher's aim is to present new facts or to help students comprehend their meaning, then a **lecture** is an appropriate teaching **method**. In other words, if medical students or residents do not know or understand something, they can walk out of your lecture knowing and understanding what they did not before.

Achievement of higher level knowledge objectives requires a more active method of teaching. If you want learners to be able to *apply*, *analyze*, *synthesize*, or *evaluate* a subject, then they have to be involved in a **group discussion**. Application requires that they use information in new situations. With analysis, they can break a subject down into its parts and, with synthesis, put it together in a new way. The highest level knowledge objective is evaluation, the ability to make judgments. Can you picture that, in a lecture, the teacher can model application, analysis, synthesis, and evaluation, but that the students need to be more actively involved for them to achieve these objectives?

Achieving each level of knowledge objectives requires achievement of the lower levels. Obviously, a student cannot comprehend what he does not know and cannot apply information not known and understood. This may explain why some group discussions fall flat. If you ask students to analyze a topic, but they do not know or comprehend the facts and have not applied or used the information in different situations, then they lack the ability to participate an analysis of the subject matter.

KROENKE'S RULES

Kurt Kroenke, who teaches in the Department of Medicine at the Brooke Army Medical Center, has suggested ten ways in which **lectures** commonly waver and could improve (1984):

1. Don't be complete.

    > Give them the rules, a few pearls that will make the lecture both memorable and applicable.... Only a good teacher can exclude the chaff and, relying on experience the audience may lack, point out not all that is possible, but rather what is probable and practical.

2. Don't mention anything once.

    Tell them what you're going to say, say it, and tell them what you said…. That which you reiterate educates.

3. Don't restate. Create.

    Too often the lecture resembles a talking review article. It's as if the listeners were a jury to be convinced rather than an audience to be educated and, yes, entertained.

4. Don't be democratic.

    Lectures require leadership…. Just as committee meetings deteriorate without an agenda, so too lectures require a format and a speaker at the center stage.

5. Don't apologize.

    Too often we hear, "I apologize for this rather busy slide," or "Forgive me for keeping you beyond the hour," or "Bear with me as we go through this detail." Busy slides should be deleted; overtime should be eliminated; complicated concepts should be simplified.

6. Don't talk about molehills to mountaineers.

    Don't offer the specialist a telescopic view and the generalist a microscopic dissection…. Talk to family practitioners on "Chest Pain," internists on "Controversies in Unstable Angina," and cardiologists on "Aortic Balloon Assist Pump for the Management of Refractory Angina."

7. Don't extemporize. Organize.

    An ad lib presentation is both superficial and desultory. Furthermore, the facts themselves are but one element in a good lecture. Repetition, selectivity, creativity, leadership, and proper choice of topics all require careful preparation.

8. Don't confess. Profess.

    Personal experience, expert opinion, imperfect answers to unanswered questions, the anecdote that illuminates, the memorable example—in these, the lecture complements the literature.

9. Don't dwell. Don't defer.

    More than five minutes in a one–hour talk is a long time. The speaker should always feel an urge to move on…. Deferring a message also can be deleterious. Mentioning a point in passing only to say, "I'll come back to that later," leads our attention astray from the present subject.

10. Start and finish.

    The germane anecdote, the story that comes naturally, the consummate cartoon—these are appropriate. Don't try too hard.

LEARNING

I hear and I forget. I see and I remember. I do and I understand.

According to Roget's College Thesaurus, learning is the antonym of teaching! Most teachers, including myself, prefer to see **teaching** and learning as a two–part process. In the Introduction, learning was described as the acquisition of information, but before it can take place, there must be interest. Teaching is the process of helping students to acquire information and creating the necessary interest that must first exist.

If this book had been written in the nineteenth century with the aim of helping to educate physicians for the twentieth–century, it would have been appropriate to quote the educational reformer John Dewey, who wrote in 1896 that, "Learning is problem solving or intelligent action in which the person continually evaluates his experience in the light of its foreseen and unforeseen consequences…learning is not simply acquisition, but a moment of experience out of which emerges redefined purposes, new evaluations, and action in the sense of continued growth" (Ratner 1939).

A century later, this concept of learning remains relevant. Learning is more than acquisition of information. For learning to last there must be a personal transformation and evaluation of the information so that it can be used and changed in the future (Bruner). This is the kind of learning that will educate physicians for the twenty–first century. By learning, I mean the ability to modify behavior in response to experience; in this framework, memory is the capacity to act upon what has been learned. The seventeenth–century French nobleman and social critic, La Rochefoucauld, said that everyone complains about the badness of his memory, no one his judgment. Yet, judgment affects memory and learning. When we judge a situation as not personally important, we stop paying attention. The technical term for this is "habituation," meaning we no longer judge the stimulus as worth attending to. Here I am reminded of the anesthetist I once knew…he put the whole class to sleep.

Learning can be described in terms of instructional **objectives** which define what the learners are expected to achieve (Bloom *et al.*). There are cognitive objectives which state achievement of **knowledge**, affective objectives which state **attitudinal change**, and psychomotor objectives which state attainment of **skills**. Often, medical teachers use these objectives to evaluate their learners. Since we are interested in rating medical students, it is appropriate to ask: What did the student learn? How much? At what level? However, we also should ask: How did the student learn? What resources were used? How efficient was the learning? These concerns with process, as well as with outcome, are important if our goal is to create life–long learners (Whitman 1981b).

LEARNING VECTOR

Thomas C. King, a professor of thoracic surgery at Columbia University College of Physicians and Surgeons, believes that the overriding purpose of education is to make the learner independent of any need for a teacher (1983). Dr. King contends that anything you do to build dependency is bad, and anything you do as a teacher to build independence is good. Thus, he concludes that the teacher as an information–giver is performing an immoral act! While I find his comments thought–provoking, it seems more practical to me to give a lot of direction to beginners and to gradually withdraw direction as the learner advances.

For example, when teaching a medical procedure, the teacher might wish to start with a demonstration and then let the learner do it. The learner will work first under close supervision and then be monitored less closely before doing it with minimal assistance. From the learner's view, this four–step approach is (1) observation, (2) practice, (3) performance on a leash, and (4) performance with a para-chute.

Frank Stritter, the Director of the Office of Research and Development for Education in the Health Professions at the University of North Carolina, is a creative educational specialist who has devised an incremental approach to professional education. This model, known as the "learning vector," is based on the assumption that clinical instruction can influence a learner's professional development in a linear or stepwise fashion and posits an approach to instruction in which the clinical instructor modifies his instruction based on the level of the student's ability. For learners at a lower level of ability to handle a clinical situation, the clinical teacher should provide *dependent* teaching strategies, and for those at higher levels of ability, the clinical teacher should provide as much *independence* as possible (Stritter 1986).

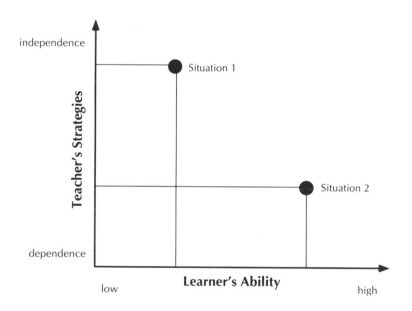

This model can provide clinical teachers with a way to analyze their medical student or resident interactions. If a student seems *anxious* (Situation 1), this may be a clue that you are providing too much independence. You may have over–estimated this person's ability to handle a patient encounter. Thus, it would be productive to modify your clinical teaching strategies to provide more dependence on you. Of course, the student may be under–confident and needs to be pushed. On the other hand, if a resident seems *frustrated* (Situation 2), this may be a clue that you are providing too much dependence. You may have under–estimated this person's ability to handle a patient encounter. Thus, it would be productive to modify your clinical teaching strategies to provide more independence from you. Of course, the resident may be over–confident and needs to be restrained.

When medical students and residents appear anxious or frustrated, a major challenge of clinical teaching is to determine whether your clinical teaching strategies should be modified to accommodate the needs of the learner or whether your initial assessment was correct and the learner needs to change his self–perception. This challenge of clinical teaching underlines the need to constantly assess the level of learner. Although some clinical teachers think that instruction equals clinical teaching, the fact is that the **preceptor's agenda** should comprise both assessment and instruction.

By and large, I believe that clinical teachers can assess the level of their learners. For example, an intern in an outpatient clinic wants to prescribe an oral hypoglycemic for a non–insulin dependent diabetic 53–year–old woman. The woman, whose mother died of a "bad heart," read in *Reader's Digest* that those pills can cause heart attacks. The intern seeks your counsel. Can you picture how a low ability versus high ability intern would approach you for help?

Nevertheless, sometimes your assessment may be wrong. There is only one strategy to resolve a disparity between your perception of a learner's clinical ability and his self–perception: two–way dialogue. If your learners seem either anxious from too little supervision or frustrated by too much, the best way to resolve the issue is for the two of you to discuss the matter. Matching teaching strategies to a learner's ability is the key to effective clinical teaching because people learn the most when there is *optimal stress*. Less learning occurs when there is too little or too much **stress**.

What makes clinical teaching particularly difficult is that, when asked to recall a memorable learning incident, most faculty relate a situation in which they had too much responsibility. Yet, as physicians responsible for patient care, they cannot in good conscience let students and residents get in over their heads. It takes a creative clinical teacher to balance the educational and service needs of a teaching hospital or ambulatory care center.

LECTURE

The lecture is a **method** of teaching in which the teacher plays an active role and, relatively speaking, the learner is passive. Planning and presenting lectures can provide an excellent opportunity to be creative. Obviously, lectures should be **useful** in that the information is scientifically sound and up–to–date. But, they also can be **novel** when teachers reveal information not available elsewhere. This occurs when medical teachers make use of their clinical and research experience (see **Kroenke's Rules**).

Medical students and residents frequently complain about lectures, deservedly so. Many medical lectures are boring, befuddling, or timewasting (Whitman in Edwards and Marier, editors, 1988). Although some medical school faculty assume that I am opposed to lectures, I am not. I am only opposed to bad ones. I strongly agree with the editors of *Change Magazine* who wrote in their *Guide to Effective Teaching*: "Nothing is worse than a poor lecture, disorganized and badly delivered. But nothing is more effective than a good lecture, combining substance with showmanship" (1978).

According to studies, the most important qualities of a good lecture are (McLeish 1976):

1.   systematic organization

2.   ability to encourage thought

3.   ability to explain clearly

4.   enthusiastic attitude toward the subject

5.   expert knowledge

These qualities also were identified in a study of medical school **teaching award winners** (Whitman and Ferrey 1986). I would add that effective lecturing begins by recognizing what you can and cannot accomplish. Basically, lower level **knowledge** objectives can be achieved in a lecture. Audience members can leave a lecture knowing facts they did not know before and they can gain a new understanding of these facts. As an example of basic knowledge or facts, one aim of a lecture to third–year medical students on a medicine clerkship might be for them to be able to recall the ranges of normal vital signs for various adult age groups. This relatively low level **objective** may be necessary to accomplish a second aim of the lecture, that they be able to discuss the physiology involved with vital signs, which is an example of a comprehension objective. Higher level objectives such as application of the information to new situations and analysis of the subject matter would require students to be more involved in their learning than is possible in a lecture. Perhaps a **group discussion** would be the appropriate teaching method.

Knowledge and comprehension, achievable in lectures, are interrelated because facts are best learned and remembered when they are *known*, *understood*, and *have meaning*. In a review of the educational psychology literature,

Higbee found that, "One of the determinants of how easy something is to learn is how meaningful it is to the learner. If it doesn't make sense, it will be hard to learn; the more meaningful it is, the easier it will be to learn" (1977, p. 37). The spirit of this "principle of meaningfulness" was captured by the physicist Ernest Rutherford, who believed that he had not completed a discovery until he was able to explain it to someone else (Highet 1950). It is this spirit that creative teachers bring to lectures. How can I make the material understandable to others?

Creative teachers also use **techniques** of teaching to attract and maintain the attention of students. Even when lecturing to large groups, it is possible to involve them with **questioning**, **brainstorming**, and **problem solving**. If a lecture is all "I talk, you listen," then it will be difficult to overcome the student passivity inherent in the lecture method. In a lecture on the epidemiology of tuberculosis, one teacher used the brainstorming technique to ask why TB incidence rates may be rising in the United States. By inviting as many responses as possible, the student–generated list looked like this:

- less government funding for screening

- more homeless people

- public apathy

- changes in the medical school curriculum

- increased immigration of refugees from third–world countries

- increased U.S. travel to third world countries

- emergence of drug resistant mutants

Generating this list took five minutes. Then the lecturer reviewed these ideas and made comments.

Often demonstrations can be arranged to highlight key points in a lecture. In a lecture on the biological mechanisms of chronic pain, the teacher brought into the classroom a patient for students to question. Even though this was a class of one hundred medical students, the teacher was able to manage the process so that students felt involved (see **physiology chicken coop**).

When I lecture on the subject of lecturing, I try to get audience members involved by asking them why I finish my lectures five minutes early. They usually come up with many good ideas, including that it improves my student evaluations and leaves time for questions. Often, they identify my real reason, which is to "leave 'em wanting more." In other words, since it is not possible to "teach it all," why give the impression of even trying? Why not let people feel a little cheated? An implicit objective of every lecture should be to motivate people to want to learn more. If you are creative, you probably could generate several ways to convey this message to your learners.

THE LECTURE PARADOX

In *The School Book*, Postman and Weingartner (1973) observed that a school is successful when its activities are *student* activities. Unfortunately, more often it is the teachers who do most of the writing, talking, and thinking: "Students take notes, which is a hell of an activity for training stenographers, but not much good for anything else." Certainly students take a lot of notes in their first two years of medical school. Are we training stenographers? (see **note–taking**)

The emphasis on transmitting information is a **criticism of medical education**, and some medical schools, including McMasters, Southern Illinois University, and Harvard, have replaced **lectures** with **problem–based**

teaching. For medical schools that continue to rely heavily upon the lecture method, Dr. LeRoy Kuehl, a professor of Biochemistry at the University of Utah School of Medicine, has identified a paradox that "compromises even the most carefully prepared lecture delivered by the most charismatic and skillful instructor."

THE PARADOX*

Three students on the door did knock;
With their Professor they would talk.
He welcomed them most cordially;
Asked: what could their problem be?
And in the office of that Saint,
They laid before him this complaint:
Your course falls short, you can't deny,
Since lecture notes you don't supply.
So all we do in your class,
Is take dictation, notes amass.
Preoccupied with pen and ink,
We have no time to learn nor think.
Your pearls of wisdom, priceless quotes
Slip by while we sit taking notes.
The good Professor promised this,
That they'd have lecture notes forthwith.
Six days he toiled and evenings too,
And when his task was finally through
Then all his lectures without fail
Were written up in great detail,
And basic concepts were defined,
Because they were all <u>underlined</u>.

Next year came students as before
To knock upon that good man's door;
To tell him how he was remiss,
And now their grievance read like this:
In lecture, everything you say
Is in the course notes anyway.
And since we all know how to read,
Of hearing you there is little need.
We could as well remain at home
And learn the subject on our own.
Could you not tell us something new
That isn't in the handouts too?
The good Professor promised this:
To remedy the flaw forthwith.
Three days he toiled and evenings too,
And when his task was finally through,
He added data and more quotes,
And minor points and anecdotes
To supplement and underscore
The topics that he'd taught before.

Next year the students came to bleat:
His lecture notes were incomplete.
For much of what he did expound,
Could nowhere in the notes be found.
Although this caused him much chagrin,
Soon to their braying he gave in,
And once again without delay
He wrote down all that he would say.

And to the old notes this was added—
His outline now was quite padded.

When yet another year had passed
And he thought he'd found peace at last,
There welled a cry from student throats
That all he did was read his notes.
The poor Professor paced the hall
Feeling like a ping–pong ball.

Thus year by year his lectures grew,
And longer were his outlines too.
And students found to their distress
They had to master an excess
Of obscure facts, minute detail;
Of information dry and stale.
A situation that attained
All because they had complained.
The moral is easy to observe:
Students get what they deserve.

LITERATURE AND MEDICINE

One creative outlet for medical teachers is the use of
literature to teach medicine. For example, Dr. David E. Ness
at the University of Pennsylvania conducts a seminar course
using the **group discussion** method to increase medical
student sensitivity to doctor–patient relationships. The

following stories and excepts from novels dealing in some way with doctor–patient interactions were chosen for their thought–provoking value:

1. "The Use of Force," William Carlos Williams

2. *Of Human Bondage*, chapter 85, W. Somerset Maugham

3. "The Horse Dealer's Daughter," D.H. Lawrence

4. "A Doctor's Visit," Anton Chekhov

5. "Ward Six," Jessamyn West

6. "The Condemned Librarian," Ivan Turgenev

7. "A Country Doctor," John Updike

Students reported that, although these works of literature were not written to instruct about the topic of doctor–patient relationships, the reading and discussion of these stories made them more aware of the feelings and thoughts that come together when doctors and patients interact.

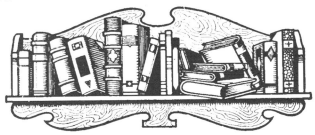

MENTOR

In my career I have profited enormously from the interactions I have had with those who served as my mentors. Such relationships were important to my own intellectual and professional development (Robert Petersdorf, President of the Association of American Medical Colleges, 1990).

Medical teachers should try to establish **professional intimacy** with *all* medical students and residents so that they can become positive **role models** for *some*. They also should consider becoming a mentor to *one or two* learners. Not all teachers become mentors, and not all medical students or residents have one. In considering the mentor's role, we recognize that the relationship between a mentor and his protégé is the ultimate teacher–student interaction.

The literature on mentoring is written almost exclusively in the male gender because traditionally women have had few mentors, male or female, and female mentors are scarce. As more women enter medical school, and ultimately become medical school faculty, this is changing. As described in the male tradition, Levinson (1978) identified several functions of the mentor which should be considered for men and women entering the field of medicine:

> He may act as a teacher to enhance the young man's skills and intellectual development. Serving as sponsor, he may use his influence to facilitate the young man's entry and advancement. He may be a host and guide, welcoming the initiate into a new occupational and social world and acquainting him with its values, customs, resources, and cast of characters. Through his own virtues, achievements, and way of living, the mentor may be an exemplar that the protégé can admire and seek to emulate. He may provide counsel and moral support in time of stress. The mentor has another critical function...developmentally the most critical one: to support and facilitate the realization of the Dream (p. 98).

Dr. R. William Betcher is a psychiatrist who was a clinical psychologist before entering medical school. As a medical student at Harvard Medical School he wrote *A Student Guide to Medical School: Study Strategies, Mnemonics, Personal Growth* (1985). In this helpful book, he recommends medical students stay in touch with their dream of being a doctor and try to reconcile their life structure to the dream, not the other way around. Mentors can play a key role in helping medical students by believing in them and in their dreams.

In a study conducted at the Medical College of Wisconsin, Kirsling and Kochar (1990) found that mentoring was a self–perpetuating phenomenon: faculty who have had mentors become mentors. They identified benefits to the protégé to include reduction of personal stress, personal growth and development, and career advancement. Based upon my own career development, I strongly endorse their conclusion:

> ...measures to enhance the growth of mentor activity between faculty and residents should be encouraged.... Increased mentor activity would likely improve communication between the housestaff and faculty, increase morale, and foster a more cooperative spirit among residents and faculty (p. 273).

METAPHORS

Judith Best, a professor of political science, encourages teachers to be more creative in the use of metaphors. In describing the metaphorical technique, she explains:

> The word metaphor comes from a Greek word that means to transfer. A metaphor

transfers meaning; it extends, stretches, twists the meaning of words so that they apply to other objects, actions, or situations than those to which they originally applied (1984, p. 165).

Metaphors can help teachers expand their view of the **teacher's role**. For example, Socrates spoke of the teacher as midwife to students pregnant with ideas. Best uses the metaphor of the teacher as a scout, who having previously traveled a path, comes back to lead the way. Is there a metaphor that describes your role as teacher? In faculty development workshops, I have heard teachers describe their role as Jehovah who breathes a soul into the clod, or the sower of seeds that fall sometimes on fertile soil, sometimes on soil that is barren. One medical school teacher referred to memory as a patchwork quilt or a pointilist painting, neither one ever quite finished (Stone 1989).

In a survey of **teaching award winners**, a medical student and I asked what metaphors they used to help students learn and remember key points (Whitman and Ferrey 1986). Here are some examples:

- Bursae function to reduce friction is like holding a partially filled balloon, whose lining is coated with oil, between your palms and moving it back and forth. There is no wear and tear on the skin of your palms.

- A cytotoxic T–cell is a Mafia cell that gives the kiss of death to a foreign or virus–infected cell.

- Interferon is a molecular Paul Revere alerting cells that "a virus is coming."

- An ocular melanoma is shaped like a mushroom.

Personal physicians think about the numerators of life and epidemiologists the numerators and the denominators.

The metaphorical technique includes similes, allegories, **anecdotes**, stories, and comparisons that are aimed at getting minds moving. Are there metaphors that can help students learn and remember what you teach? Related to metaphors are mnemonics, devices to help students remember facts. For example, did you learn the eight bones in the wrist with the mnemonic, "Never lower Tillie's pants; grandmother might come home"? While mnemonics aid memory, metaphors increase understanding.

METHODS

Methods of teaching describe the relationship between teachers and learners (Whitman 1981a). As can be seen in the figure, in the **teaching learning–process**, there are two potential actors, the teacher and the learner, and two possible modes of behavior, active or passive. When the teacher is active in a classroom setting, but the students are relatively passive, this is a **lecture**. When both the teacher and the learners are active, this is a **group discussion**. This difference between the lecture and group discussion was noted by one professor who commented that, "The true difference is one of method. In discussions students ideally teach themselves. In lectures teachers teach them" (Segal).

Of course, much medical education occurs outside the classroom, in the clinical setting. When the teacher is active, but the learners are relatively passive, this is a **preceptorship**. When the teacher is more passive, and the learners are active, this is a tutorial. I am using the terms "preceptorship" and "tutorial" in a generic sense, recognizing that some medical schools call clinical rotations in private practices preceptorships regardless of the relationship between the teacher and the learner. Also, I recognize that a clinical experience may slide between preceptorship and tutorial depending upon the student or resident's ability to handle a specific patient encounter.

	Active Teacher	Passive Teacher
Active Learner	group discussion	tutorial
Passive Learner	lecture / preceptorship	

Lecturing is the most common method of teaching in the classrooms of medical schools. In fact, David E. Rogers, former President of the Robert Wood Johnson Foundation, observed that medical students felt they were being lectured to death. His comment stimulated Dr. Thomas L. Schwenk, a former Robert Wood Johnson Fellow in Faculty Development and currently Chairman of Family Practice at the University of Michigan Medical School, and me to write *A Handbook for Group Discussion Leaders: Alternatives to Lecturing Medical Students to Death.*

We are not opposed to lectures, provided they are aimed at the appropriate instructional **objectives**, *i.e.,* helping students learn new facts and/or increase understanding of those facts. However, if your **knowledge** objectives are higher, *i.e.*, teaching students to apply, analyze, synthesize, or evaluate information, or if your objective is **attitudinal change**, then the group discussion method is more appropriate.

Of course, even if the teaching method is appropriately matched to the instructional objectives, it must be effectively implemented. Just as not every topic is best addressed with a group discussion, not every teacher possesses a ready set of interpersonal behaviors that will predict success as a group discussion leader. Some medical school teachers, whose repertoire of facts and entertaining style of delivery have led to great success as a lecturer, fail miserably in attempting to lead a group discussion dealing with the same topic.

Conversely, some faculty who excel in leading a group discussion become nervous and awkward in front of a lecture audience. The great nineteenth century biologist, Thomas Huxley, recalled that his first lecture "made at twenty–seven before one of the glittering and monumentally starched audiences of the Royal Institution, was begun in terror and concluded in the earnest conviction of intelligibility" (Irvine):

> When I took a glimpse into the room and saw it full of faces, I did feel most amazingly uncomfortable. I can now understand what it is to be going to be hanged and nothing but the necessity of the case prevented me from running away.

Medical faculty also differ in their clinical teaching strengths. Some instructors prefer the more active teaching role of the preceptorship and especially enjoy the close supervision that might be appropriate for medical students. Others feel more comfortable in the less active teaching role of the tutorial, preferring the more collegial relationship typical of working with residents. In either case it is important to accurately assess the needs of the learner so that teaching strategies are suitably matched. As described in Stritter's **Learning Vector**, learners who feel they are given too much leeway may feel anxious, and those who are too closely monitored may feel frustrated.

MORNING REPORT

At morning report, there are often strong conflicts between patient care needs and educational **objectives**. Do any of the following scenarios look familiar?

1.   The attending is notorious for arriving late and leaving early. Knowing this, the admitting resident presents the most complicated patient first. As the resident finishes, the attending, who has arrived in the middle of the presentation, makes a few superficial remarks and abruptly leaves.

2.   During a resident's presentation of a patient admission, practically every resident is paged to the telephone for at least part of the report, so that by the end no one is able to discuss the entire case. The larger group deteriorates into a two–way discussion between the admitting resident and the attending physician, with the rest of the ward team looking bored and wanting to get on to their patient rounds.

3.   After the case presentation is finished, the chief resident and the attending physician debate a point that no one else cares about. As they discuss this issue, others leave the room one–by–one as they are paged (or jolt their beepers).

4.   A complex patient is presented and the attending physician explains how to best manage the case. As the team prepares to visit the patient, he asks whether there are any questions. They all shake their heads, "No."

According to Schwenk and Whitman (1987) the easiest way to fail to meet the educational objectives of morning report is to take so long that the residents and students check out, physically or mentally. Thus, it is important to use an approach that highlights important points rather than tries to cover all points. They recommend no more than fifteen minutes for most new patients, allowing perhaps twenty to thirty minutes for a more complex case.

One **criticism of medical education** is that clinical teachers do not preach what they practice! Jerome Kassirer, who was recognized at the 1989 annual meeting of the Association of American Medical Colleges as one of the nation's outstanding medical teachers, asks why we present the entire patient data base to a morning report team before asking them to **problem solve**? He recommends that team members ask for specific items from the patient's history, physical examination, and laboratory results, thereby simulating the process followed by the admitting resident.

MOTIVATION

Some desire is necessary to keep life in motion (Samuel Johnson).

While it is mainly the student's responsibility to become motivated and teachers cannot make students learn, teachers can promote learning by helping students become motivated to learn. Motivation is the *interaction between personal and environmental factors*, and teachers definitely influence the medical school environment. For example, teachers can create a physical environment that encourages sharing and reduces barriers between teachers and students. So, in small classes, the teacher can arrange the chairs in a semi–circle rather than in rows, and in a large class, the teacher can move about the room rather than stand behind a podium. In the clinical setting, attending physicians can foster a team approach to medical problem solving, welcoming participation from all members of the team.

Teachers can also create a social environment that reduces barriers to learning. Do you ask questions for the sake of stimulating students to think or do you practice the art of **pimping**, ridding students and residents of needless self esteem? Do learners feel free to ask questions? Do they feel free to say, "I don't know," or do they play the "**pretend to know game**"?

Being conversational and reducing the psychological distance between teachers and students also influence student motivation. Richard Wallen, an educational psychologist, has coined the phrase "psychological size" as a convenient label to describe the impact of one person upon another. Psychological size interferes with open dialogue when one party is psychologically bigger than another (Fuhrmann and Grasha 1983). Whereas pimping "inculcates the intern with profound and abiding respect for his attending physician" (Brancati), teachers who want to motivate students and residents treat them as colleagues.

Teachers can motivate students by showing that they understand the students' position and by respecting them. They come to your classes wondering what lies ahead. You can let them know from the start what major issues will be explored and what important questions will be asked. They come to your clinical rotations wondering what they will be responsible for and what clinical skills they will be performing. You can let them know your expectations and what it takes to be successful.

The importance of establishing a supportive learning environment in medical education was emphasized by Skeff and colleagues who observed that the tone of the teaching setting is a key element of learning and includes whether medical students are stimulated and attentive and whether they feel comfortable to participate and reveal their strengths and weaknesses.

The **feedback** teachers give students and residents about their performance can be motivating or de–motivating, depending on how it is given. If feedback is demeaning or belittling, many students will become defensive. If it is constructive, they will be grateful and put energy into improvement. Also, positive feedback for good performance is motivating. During a presentation at the 1986 annual meeting of the Association of Program Directors in Surgery, I shared with these residency directors my perception that surgery residents get negative feedback even when they deserve positive. I asked them whether this was the case. What do you think they said? Overwhelmingly, they confirmed this was true. Furthermore, they told me it was a good educational practice: "It keeps residents on their toes!" Frankly, my understanding of human behavior is that when people do a good job and are told so, they feel motivated to do an even better job.

Of course, the feedback students and residents give to faculty about their teaching also can be motivating or de–motivating. Not all faculty care what their students and residents think about their teaching (see **student ratings**), but many do care. Furthermore, the motivation of some faculty depends upon the motivation of the students and residents, and the quality of their teaching depends upon the quality of their students. If they have enthusiastic students, their teaching is inspired, and if they have uninterested students, their teaching languishes (Tiberius *et al.* 1989).

Whether you believe in carrots or sticks, motivation should be your concern because the formula for student learning can be expressed as *motivation times ability*. Given two medical students with equal knowledge and skills, the one with the higher motivation will learn more. Although it is up to students to be motivated, how teachers teach can help motivate or de–motivate them. Related to motivation is the level of **stress**. Simply stated, people learn less when there is either too little or too much stress.

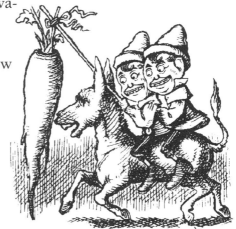

MULTI–INSTRUCTOR COURSES

Many medical school courses, especially in the basic sciences, are taught by multiple instructors. Studies of **student ratings** demonstrate that their evaluations of single–instructor courses are reliable. To what extent can students form judgments of teaching in multi–instructor courses? In a study of student ratings of a multi–instructor course at the University of Washington School of Medicine, Irby and colleagues (1977) demonstrated that student ratings obtained immediately after each lecture and at the end of the course were sensitive to differences in teaching ability among thirteen faculty and were highly correlated, although students did report some loss of specific recall ability.

Because of the stability of ratings, end–of–course ratings are adequate for evaluating individual faculty and the overall course (summative evaluation). However, end–of–lecture ratings would be more appropriate for faculty and course improvement (formative evaluation) because of the greater specificity of student comments. The use of student ratings for the purpose of formative evaluation in a multi–instructor course at the University of Arizona College of Medicine was studied by Stillman and colleagues (1983) who found that end–of–lecture immediate feedback was appreciated by students and faculty. The results of their two–year study demonstrated that, not only did instructors who presented the same lectures during both years improve, but the overall course evaluation improved as well. Also, instructors in the second year who did not teach in the first year received significantly higher ratings than those who gave the same lectures the previous year, possibly because the evaluation system helped to weed out weaker instructors.

MYTHS OF MEDICAL EDUCATION

Dr. Stephen Abrahamson, one of the pioneers in the field of medical faculty development, describes four myths typically heard during discussions of medical teaching (1989):

1. *"It doesn't matter which curriculum a medical school uses."*

    A more acceptable statement might be that, given how bright and gifted the students are, certain curricular variations may not make a significant difference for many students. But, if we are truly educating physicians for the twenty–first century, our curriculum had better take into account how medicine will be practiced.

2.   *"Our educational goals are clear to us and our students."*

Although faculty and students may have a broad sense of their school's goals and **objectives**, there may not be a clear sense of direction. For example, often I wonder whether teaching is a product or by-product of the medical school.

3.   *"First students have to learn the vocabulary."*

The McMaster Medical School pioneered a curriculum that has been adapted by other medical schools, including Southern Illinois University and Harvard. It demonstrates that students can learn the vocabulary of medicine while they engage in medical **problem solving.** During my grand rounds on medical education at the Hershey Medical Center, a physician in the back row challenged me on this point. I asked him whether English was his second language. Surprised, he replied, "Of course not." Then I asked how he learned to speak it so well.

4.   *"Students need my lectures to learn the material."*

Different students learn in different ways, and even a given student may learn in different ways at different times. Since **teaching** means helping another person learn, a more acceptable statement may be that some students, some of the time, are helped by my **lectures**.

MYTHS OF TEACHING

According to the late Kenneth Eble, an award–winning teacher at the University of Utah and specialist in the field of faculty development, there are several myths of teaching (1988, pp.11–12) including:

1. Teaching is not doing.

2. Teaching is not a performing art.

3. Teaching should exclude the personality.

4. Students' "worst" teachers now will become their "best" teachers later.

5. The popular teacher is a **bad teacher**.

6. Teachers are born and not made.

7. Good and bad teaching cannot be identified.

8. Research is complementary to teaching.

9. Teaching a subject matter requires only that one knows it.

10. Teaching is not a profession.

THE NEW MEXICO EXPERIMENT

On morning rounds Dr. Elliott and I found our patient gasping for air, frantic. She was an 84–year–old Hispanic woman who spoke little English. Although Dr. Elliott tried to explain to her what a respirator was, I think neither she nor I was prepared for the intubation. After she was on the breathing machine and had slipped into a drugged sleep, I went to our rural hospital's small library down the hall to study the basis of what I had just seen—the anatomy of the larynx and bronchi and how arterial blood gases reflect acid–base balance (Kaufman et al. 1989).

This first–year medical student is participating in an experimental curriculum implemented at the University of New Mexico School of Medicine in 1977. In order to equip its graduates with skills in self–directed, lifelong learning and to motivate them to practice primary care in rural settings,

New Mexico introduced three innovations in its medical curriculum:

1. **Problem–based teaching** is used to promote understanding and retention of medical knowledge.

2. **Student–centered learning** is used to help students take responsibility for their own education.

3. Community health experiences, including four months in the first year, are used to immerse students in primary care settings (see **apprenticeship**).

The program evaluation after ten years demonstrates positive results, including comparison of students in the traditional and experimental programs (see **Harvard's New Pathway**).

NOTE–TAKING

Medical teachers often ask me whether they should encourage students to take notes during lectures. On one hand, they want students to listen, rather than write. On the other hand, they are concerned that most of what students hear will be forgotten if they do not take notes (see **lecture paradox**). The solution lies in giving students a handout. Handouts can serve two functions: storage and encoding (Divesta and Gray 1972). By *storage*, we mean providing students a record of the lecture which they can study later. Of course, you could provide a complete transcript of the talk, providing complete storage, but this would encourage passive listening or even non–attendance. *Encoding* refers to the process of students converting the teacher's words into their own, encouraging active listening. But, some students find it difficult to listen and write at the same time and do not take good notes.

In order to study the effects of three types of lecture notes on learning, medical educators at the University of Texas at San Antonio used three types of handouts in a lecture on fibrositis and hypertension (Russell *et al.* 1983). The *comprehensive* handout was very detailed, containing a nearly word–for–word transcript of the lecture including all the tables and figures from the slides. The *partial* handout consisted of an outline with key tables and figures. The *skeletal* handout had only a very brief outline with ample space for note–taking. Based on student test results, they found that the partial handout was the best compromise, balancing the storage advantages of the comprehensive handout and the encoding advantages of the skeletal.

NOVELTY

Creative teachers are both novel and **useful**. By novel, I mean using methods and techniques that awaken the learner. Teachers who are novel find ways to create interest in their material and motivate the learners to want to learn. Unfortunately, some medical teachers take the view summarized by Mager and Pipe as "they really oughta wanna." I am left with the impression that these faculty see themselves as "live textbooks," presenting as much informa-tion as possible in the allotted time...often going "overtime" to cover additional material. In one physiology lecture, the teacher already had spilled over into the ten–minute break, and the next teacher had entered the lecture hall, waiting for his turn to speak. The physiologist could see that students were no longer listening, so he said, "Hang in there. I will stop in five more minutes." Of course, by now, most students had stopped learning.

How can you create interest and motivate learners? How can you stimulate adults to learn? Keller (1987) highlighted the importance of *attention, relevance, confidence,* and *satisfaction.* In order to capture the attention of students and to make what they learn relevant to them, ask yourself, "How can I make this material valuable and stimulating to my students? What prior knowledge and experience can I build upon?" In order to help students feel confident and satisfied with their performance, ask yourself, "How can I help students succeed and give them as much control as possible? What activities will produce student involvement and participation?"

Teachers who are novel create a learning climate that encourages students to become involved in their own education. The importance of this learning climate was emphasized by an outstanding medical teacher, Kelley Skeff, who identified learner involvement, stimulation, and respect as key elements of clinical teaching. Of course, some teachers believe that avoidance of boredom is primarily the student's responsibility. Although you cannot make students want to learn, I do not think the desire for knowledge is their responsibility alone. After all, no matter how interested the students are at the beginning of a class or clinical rotation, it is possible to bore them if you try hard enough. In this regard, the late poet, John Ciardi, once quipped that there are no dull teachers—only dull people in classrooms impersonating teachers (see **boring teachers**).

Techniques you might cultivate to become a real teacher, rather than an impersonator, include **questioning, brainstorming, demonstrating, role playing,** and **problem solving**. These techniques comprise a repertoire for the creative teacher.

OBJECTIVES

The connectedness of things is the most important goal of education (Mark VanDoren).

Most medical teachers are familiar with instructional objectives. Objectives are statements which describe what the learner is expected to achieve as a result of instruction. Because they direct attention to the student and the types of behavior he should exhibit, sometimes these statements are called "behavioral" objectives. Behavioral objectives were first used in World War II when the United States faced the tremendous educational challenge of training millions of civilians to become military personnel. In the 1950s, this approach to education was applied to public schools and later to colleges and universities.

By the 1960s, most health professional schools were translating their educational intentions into "instructional objectives." In the 1960s and 70s, many workshops were conducted to teach faculty how to write instructional objectives. In 1971, when I was an instructor in the Department of Community Dentistry at the New Jersey Dental School, I attended such a workshop and was given a copy of *Preparing Instructional Objectives* by Robert Mager. Thousands of other faculty have been given copies over the past thirty years. The book is only sixty pages long and has wide margins. Never has a book with more white space had a greater impact on American education!

Another great influence on the instructional objectives movement was the work done by committees under the direction of Bloom (1956) to classify cognitive objectives and Krathwohl (1964) to classify affective objectives. *Cognitive* objectives describe intellectual outcomes and include, in ascending order of difficulty: knowledge, comprehension, application, analysis, synthesis, and evaluation. *Affective* objectives include attitudes, values, and beliefs. The classification of *psychomotor* objectives that describe skills and procedures was not completed until the 1970s (Gronlund 1978).

The movement toward objectives has not been without its critics. Some teachers counseled against the use of objectives because they felt that emphasis on objectives would draw teachers to pedestrian, more easily–operationalized objectives rather than higher level, difficult to measure goals (Popham). To be fair, it is true that faculty often write trivial objectives because objectives that describe more important learning are harder to write. Nevertheless, I support the notion that both teachers planning instruction and student participants are more effective when they know in advance what **knowledge**, **attitudinal change**, and **skills** are expected.

To avoid trivialization, faculty should be on guard against a disproportionate number of objectives written at the *basic knowledge* level that use verbs such as define, list, and recall. In addition, students should be able to demonstrate *comprehension* (discuss, describe, explain), *application* (demonstrate, interpret, predict), *analysis* (distinguish, classify, compare/contrast), *synthesis* (propose, hypothesize, diagnose), and *evaluation* (assess, justify, choose). Faculty should not avoid the affective domain of attitudes, values, and beliefs. Statements of affective outcomes include "show sensitivity to…" "accept responsibility for…" "be willing to…" and "demonstrate commitment to…".

Instructional objectives can be useful to teachers and learners when they have been thoughtfully conceived. However, when constructed solely to satisfy requirements of a school curriculum committee or external accreditation agency, objectives may be less than helpful. Personally, I like the statement prepared by faculty in my department when they prepared their first set of objectives for the Family Medicine Residency Program in 1975.

> We have defined learning objectives for several reasons. Generally, they are clear statements of an individual's performance that can be directly observed. Also they are essential for the development of the curriculum and evaluation. Instructors and chiefs of clinical services who participate in the teaching program no longer need to wonder if their efforts coincide with the objectives of the program. Perhaps the major benefit of this document will be to the resident who needs an indication of the progress he is making toward becoming a family physician (DFCM 1975).

Of course, there have been many changes in the residency program since 1975, which means that objectives have had to be modified accordingly. Perhaps the greatest benefit of preparing objectives is the focused attention given to the evolution of an educational program. T.S. Eliot, commenting on Dante's *Inferno*, described Hell as someplace where nothing connects with nothing. Instructional objectives, when thoughtfully written and periodically reviewed, help teachers and learners connect the educational process to its intended outcome.

PAP SMEAR

There are four ways in which **clinical teaching is like clinical care**. The mnemonic PAP Smear can help you remember these:

P . . . . *Problems* are solved. In clinical care, you diagnose a patient's problem and in clinical teaching you assess the learner's needs.

A . . . . *Aims* are therapeutic. In both cases, another person should be better off as a result of an interaction with you.

P . . . . *People* are funny! Patients are anxious about being embarrassed. So are medical students and residents.

S . . . . *Skills* are interchangeable. Both clinical care and clinical teaching require the same set of interactive communication skills, including attentive silence, cooperative negotiation, and the art of persuasion.

PEER TEACHING

Docendo discimus. I teach, therefore I learn.

Peer teaching refers to students teaching students in situations that are planned and directed by a teacher. In peer teaching, students learn through a variety of situations in which students work together. Most teachers know that the best way to learn something is to teach it. Thus, peer teaching provides students with the benefits traditionally enjoyed by their professors. Of course, peer teaching would not be feasible if there were no peer learning. Peer teachers are believed to benefit learners because of their closeness as peers. Here I am reminded of the eight–year–old teaching another eight–year–old how to play chess. In a few minutes, they are playing a game that we would be willing to call "chess." Yet, if a chess grand master tried to teach me how to play, unless he was an adept teacher, it would likely be a frustrating experience (Whitman 1988).

The benefit to both the peer teacher and the peer learner can be seen when medical procedures are demonstrated. The benefit to the peer teacher is expressed in the surgical dictum, "See one, do one, teach one." And, because the peer teacher has just learned the skill, he probably will teach at the right level for the learner. Experienced clinicians, like chess grand masters, may become easily frustrated or impatient (see **learning vector**) with beginners.

Peer tutoring can be an effective remedy for students in academic difficulty. For example, the University of Texas Medical Branch at Galveston implemented a peer tutoring system for students with deficient grades in basic science courses. The tutors included doctoral students in the Graduate School of Biomedical Sciences and junior and senior medical students. At the end of two terms, the mean test scores of fifty–five freshmen and sophomores in the program increased from 69 to 76 (Trevino and Eiland 1980). The University of Maryland School of Medicine also implemented a peer tutoring system to help students having difficulty with basic science courses. The tutors were sophomores, juniors, and seniors who had done well in these courses. The overall impact on students in academic difficulty was positive and the peer teachers appreciated the opportunity to review material they would need to know for National Boards (Walker–Bartnick, Berger, and Kappelman 1984).

Medical students and residents also can be helpful in counseling their peers. In turn, they help themselves by helping others. This notion is known as the "helper therapy principle." As formulated by Riessman (1965), it is clear that patients with chronic diseases benefit from helping other patients:

> An age–old therapeutic approach is the use of people with a problem to help other people who have the same problem in a more severe form. But in the use of this approach...it may be that emphasis is being placed on the wrong person in centering attention on the person receiving help. More attention might well be given the individual who needs help less, that

is, the person who is providing the assistance, because frequently it is he who improves (p. 27).

PHYSIOLOGY CHICKEN COOP

In June, 1983, the Department of Physiology at the University of Utah School of Medicine invited me to conduct a workshop on lecture skills. In part, their request was motivated by low **student ratings** of their course. In the workshop, I introduced the faculty to the **Doctor Fox** effect, which refers to the influence of a teacher's personality on student ratings of instruction. After the workshop, the Physiology faculty proposed that I give one of their lectures.

They chose the lecture on the biological mechanisms of chronic pain. Dr. Burgess, the neurophysiologist who usually gave this lecture, had been disappointed with his own efforts to teach this topic, and he was curious to see how an educational specialist would teach it. The results of this experiment were subsequently published under the title, "Dr. Fox in the Physiology Chicken Coop" (Whitman and Burgess).

To prepare for the lecture, I met with Dr. Burgess for an hour and a half. He did his best to tutor me in a subject about which I knew nothing. I then spent two hours in the medical library, reviewing my notes and reading basic textbooks. I made an interesting discovery while reading one book: I realized that the "no C receptors" in my tutorial notes were in reality the pain receptors known as "nociceptors." I drafted a lecture text and spent another hour and a half with Dr. Burgess to review the material and to make sure that I would present the material he wanted the students to learn. With this preparation, I faced one hundred freshmen medical students to lecture on a subject I had just learned myself. The students were not forewarned that I was not a subject matter expert. As far as we know, they assumed I was a faculty member from the Department of Physiology.

In this lecture, I tried to model the teaching skills recommended in my handbook for medical lectures, *There Is No Gene for Good Teaching.* For example, I stated the purpose clearly, explained the relevance of the material, highlighted key points, used a conversational manner and ended on time. In particular, I used a technique to maintain student attention: since research supports the notion that attention in a lecture begins to wane in twenty minutes, I introduced the students to a chronic pain patient at that point and let students ask her questions.

The student response to the lecture was positive. First, they applauded the patient at the end of the questioning period. Then, to the surprise of the faculty observing the lecture, they applauded me at the end of the lecture. Furthermore, this lecture received the highest student rating in the course. What was the faculty response to these findings? When I suggested that they could learn how to teach more effectively, they concluded that I should learn and teach more physiology!

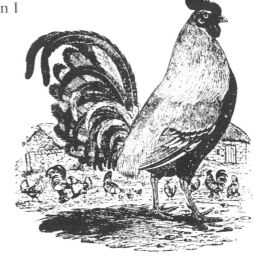

PIMPING

During the second half of 1989, participants in several workshops on clinical teaching asked me if I had seen the editorial on pimping in *JAMA*. In fact, my department chairman already had sent me a copy of this article written by Frederick L. Brancati, who teaches in the Department of Medicine at the University of Pittsburgh. With tongue–in–cheek humor, Brancati provides a primer to the fine art of pimping. According to Brancati, there are five category of pimp questions:

1. Arcane points of history that are not taught in medical school and are irrelevant to patient care, for example, "Who performed the first lumbar puncture?" Or, "How was syphilis named?"

2. Teleology and metaphysics that lie outside the realm of conventional scientific inquiry, for example, "Why are some organs paired?"

3. Exceedingly broad questions that cannot be answered completely, for example, "What role do prostaglandins play in homeostasis?" Or, "What is the differential diagnosis of a fever of unknown origin?"

4. Eponyms favored by old–timers, for example, "Where does one find the semilunar space of Traube?" Or, "Whose name is given to the dancing uvula of aortic regurgitation?"

5. Technical points of laboratory research, for example, "How active are leukocyte–activated killer cells with or without interleukin 2 against sarcoma in the mouse model?"

Although pimping may appear to be a form of the Socratic method of **questioning** students to uncover what they already know or can know (Socrates used the **metaphor** of the teacher serving as a midwife to students pregnant with ideas), the **motivation** is different. Whereas the Socratic method of questioning is intended to increase the confidence of learners, Brancati points out that pimping inculcates "a profound and abiding respect for (the) attending physician while ridding (students and residents) of needless self–esteem."

Of course, students and residents use numerous defenses against pimping. The same strategies probably were used by today's pimpers in their formative years. When being pimped, a student or resident can dodge by answering the question with a question or answering a different question. Or he can bluff an answer, which, if not called by the attending physician, can promulgate medical lies.

My major objection to pimping is that it encourages medical students and residents to play the "**pretend to know game**," in which they hide gaps in their knowledge. This game is an obstacle to the **teaching–learning process** because, if played successfully, opportunities for instruction will be missed.

PLAIN DOCTORING

Plain Doctoring is an elective, preclinical seminar at Harvard Medical School designed to introduce medical students to "the day–to–day experiences of seeing patients, the joys and frustrations of working as physicians, or grappling with (their) lives and those of their patients and their families" (Billings *et al.* 1985, p. 855). In this course, patients who have a chronic illness or an unusual life story volunteer to talk at home to visiting students. Before making these visits, the faculty and students meet to discuss useful questions. Also, short stories about doctor–patient relationships (see **literature and medicine**) are assigned. After their home visits, students discuss their observations and the reading material in a seminar.

At the end of the course, students complete a project in which they are encouraged to be creative. Projects may include photo essays on their house call, short stories and poems based on their encounter, or slide shows with recorded music. Students report electing the course to learn **humanistic behavior**. In their course evaluations, while some students express discomfort with the lack of structure, most say that the course was inspirational (see **attitudinal change**).

PLATFORM CHICANERY

The need to give information in **lectures** that could as easily be read by the students was attacked by B.F. Skinner in his novel, *Walden Two*. In that book, a member of a utopian community tells a visiting university professor:

> The lecture is the most inefficient method of diffusing culture. It became obsolete with the invention of printing. It survives only in our universities and their lay imitators, and a few other backward institutions.... Why don't you just hand printed lectures to your students? Yes, I know. Because they won't read them. A fine institution it is that must solve that problem with platform chicanery (1948, p. 42).

Is lecturing platform chicanery? The **Doctor Fox** studies support the notion that students can be fooled by a professional actor programmed to teach charismatically, but non–substantively. There is the potential abuse of the charlatan, *i.e.*, the teacher who is novel in how in teaches, but not useful in what he teaches. If I will not defend the charlatan, I hope you will not defend the pedantic bore, *i.e.*, the teacher who is useful, but not novel. Teachers who are creative are both useful and novel.

Of course, Skinner has raised an interesting question. Why lecture if the material can be read? My position is that lectures should include information not in print and information which has to be synthesized from many print sources. What information is not available in print? There are the results of your unpublished research and your clinical experience. Bringing these results and experiences into the lecture supplements what can be read by the students and makes them aware of what you do as a faculty member. If this information is relevant to student needs, then telling this information is a valuable use of you as a resource.

Synthesizing information from many sources is also a good use of you as a resource if the students lack the time, interest, or expertise to do the synthesis themselves. We know from studies of **peer teaching** that students probably would learn more if they did the synthesis and taught it to others, just as you do. But, at times, this may not be practical.

It is not platform chicanery to use lectures to help create interest in a subject and to motivate students to read on their own. Nor is it platform chicanery to present information not available or not readily available in print. Unfortunately, some medical school teachers are no more than live textbooks, imparting information that can easily be read. I support the position of J. Michael Bishop, Professor in the

Department of Microbiology and Immunology at the University of California, San Francisco, School of Medicine (winner of the 1989 Nobel Prize for Medicine):

> What are the purposes and priorities of teaching? First, to inspire. Second, to challenge. Third, and only third, to impart information (1984, p. 96).

PRECEPTOR'S AGENDA

Preceptors often express the concern that they do not know *how to teach*. However, the fact is that doctors who know how to talk with and listen to patients already have developed the skills needed to teach medical students and residents. That is why I like to say that **clinical teaching is like clinical care.** When they choose to, clinicians know how to listen, how to establish two–way communication, and how to take control of a conversation. Just as talking with patients is primarily a conversation focused on their needs, teaching medical students and residents requires determining their needs. Thus the preceptor's agenda must begin with *assessment*, which helps to bring into focus the second agenda item, *instruction*. (Whitman and Schwenk 1984).

When it comes to instruction, some preceptors are concerned that they do not know *what to teach*. Here we are concerned with three types of **learning**: knowledge, attitude, and skill. By **knowledge**, I have more in mind than information which appears in medical journals and textbooks. Of greater importance is the personal knowledge that preceptors have gained in their years of clinical practice. **Attitudinal change** is equally important in medical teaching. Preceptors have developed personal views, beliefs, and values over the years that medical students and residents may not encounter in the medical school setting. Finally, preceptors have much to offer in the teaching of **skills** because what works in the office may differ from what is taught in the medical school. Thus, preceptors are rich in their ability to teach knowledge, attitude, and skill.

However, if you are not aware of the learner's *current* knowledge, attitude, and skill, teaching may be inefficient and unproductive. That is why the preceptor's agenda begins with assessment. Through **questioning**, you can find out what the learners do and do not know so you can aim instruction toward what they do not know. The difficulty with assessing knowledge is that students and residents may feel they are being tested. Given their medical school experience, this is understandable. Many students and residents have learned how to play the "**pretend to know game**" to cover up knowledge deficiencies. As a result, a preceptor may have to explain the reason for his questioning.

Attitudes also are difficult to assess because students and residents may not want to be open with you, especially if they think you are going to be judgmental when their personal views, beliefs, and values differ from yours. Here it is important to establish a **professional intimacy** with the learner to encourage authenticity.

Assessment of skills provides a unique contribution by the preceptor because many medical students and residents are not observed interviewing patients. In fact, one **criticism of medical education** is that there is little or no observation after the sophomore patient interviewing course.

Teaching knowledge, attitude, and skill requires sharing clinical experiences, role modeling, and demonstration with opportunity for practice. Realistically, a single preceptor cannot address all learner needs. Since you cannot "teach it all" at least you can uncover needs that were unknown to the learner so he can address these elsewhere in the curriculum.

Clearly, precepting is a highly personal type of teaching. Whether the preceptor is located in a private office or in a hospital outpatient department, there will be close interaction between a teacher and learner and between the two of them and a patient. The intensity of these interactions is summarized for me by one experienced teacher who said:

> Perhaps there is no effort which is as total or
> which makes one so vulnerable as teaching.
> He who attempts it reaches beyond himself
> and senses that his best is not good enough
> (Frost).

Your "best" not only is good enough, but is essential to training physicians for the twenty–first century.

PRECEPTORSHIPS

A preceptorship is an educational experience in which a medical student or resident spends a period of time in a practice setting outside the academic medical center. Dr. Joseph Scherger, a past president of the Society of Teachers of Family Medicine and recipient of the STFM Family Doctor of the Year Award, published an article on preceptorships while still a medical student. Having experienced several preceptorships during his medical education, he noted that "too often preceptors are unaware of the responsibilities of their position and the delicate nature of their exchange with students" (1975, p. 201).

In 1975, there was little literature on preceptorships, which certainly is no longer the case. One article subsequently published identified four responsibilities: "The preceptor is role model, educational guide, career counselor and clinical consultant" (Margon 1979, p. 89). Each responsibility deserves comment.

1. One does not "prepare" to be a role model, but the responsibility is to be self–conscious enough to ask the student or resident to reflect on his behaviors. For example, the preceptor should be "honest and explicit about how he deals with uncertainty or difficult decisions, allowing the student or resident to question and adopt certain aspects as part of his own developing style" (Margon 1979, p. 90).

2. As an educational guide, the **preceptor's agenda** is to assess and instruct, just as he diagnoses and treats as a clinician. These parallel roles were described by Gil *et al.* (1981) who commented that the functions of the physician–teacher within medicine and education are the same: (a) the statement of a problem, (b) information gathering, (c) diagnostic decisions, and (d) treatment recommendations.

3. Although most clinical training occurs in hospital inpatient services, this is not the environment where most medical school graduates will spend the majority of their professional time. According to a national survey of senior medical students, sixty percent indicated that their first choice of professional activity was in the private clinical practice of medicine or in the employment of a prepaid health group (Gary 1987). One family practice preceptor commented that as a medical student, he was uncertain which specialty to pursue. He arranged for two preceptorships, one in obstetrics and gynecology and one in family medicine. These experiences were so informative and instructive that he structured the third year of his residency training along preceptorship lines in orthopedics, dermatology, obstetrics and gynecology, internal medicine, and rural family practice. In retrospect, he wrote: "These preceptors became strong **role**

models for me. To this day I see their style and attitudes mirrored in my own behavior" (Bateman 1987, p. 10).

4. As a clinical consultant, preceptors can provide a one–to–one dialogue with students and residents. In a literature review conducted by Irby (1978), the best clinical teachers (a) show that they are enthusiastic about teaching, (b) explain clinical material clearly, summarizing and emphasizing what is important to learn, and (c) demonstrate the ability to solve medical problems.

In return for providing role modeling, educational guidance, career counseling, and clinical consultation, the preceptor can benefit from the preceptorship. One preceptor commented :

> Most of all there is the inherent fun and enjoyment that comes from teaching and setting a compassionate, scholarly example for these interesting, bright future physicians.... The rewards of creative preceptorship management more than balance the efforts (Sophocles 1987, p. 14)

PRETEND TO KNOW GAME

A major obstacle to the **teaching–learning process** in the clinical setting is the "pretend to know game." Medical students and residents play this game because, in an ego–intensive environment, people hate to say "I don't know." You may have played this game when you were a student or resident, so you know its rules:

1. Avoid eye contact with the attending physician when he asks the ward team a question and you do not know the answer.

2. Nod in agreement when someone else answers a question and sounds like he knows what he is talking about.

3. Answer a question with a question if you do not know the answer.

The penalty paid when students and residents successfully play this game is that the teacher may miss an opportunity to teach. This was underscored in a poem written by the psychoanalyst, R.D. Laing (*Knots* 1970, reprinted by permission of Pantheon Books).

> There is something I don't know
> that I am supposed to know.
> I don't know *what* it is I don't know,
> and yet am supposed to know.
> And I feel I look stupid
> if I seem both not to know it
> and not know *what* it is I don't know.
> Therefore, I pretend I know it.
> This is nerve–wracking
> since I don't know what I must pretend to know.
> Therefore I pretend to know everything.
> I feel you know what I am suppose to know
> but you can't tell me what it is
> because you don't know that I don't know what it is.
> You may know what I don't know, but not
> that I don't know it.
> And I can't tell you. So you will have to
> tell me everything.

To prevent this game–playing, let your students and residents know on Day One that you know how this game is played and you do not want them playing it. Promise to make it rewarding, not punishing, when they admit what they do not know. Let them know that you might show disappointment when they do not know what you think they should know, but that your aim will be to teach, not to humiliate. When they admit what they do not know, you might tell them what they do not know or you might show them the resources they could use to find out on their own. In any case, what they do not know should be used as a stimulus for their learning, not an attempt to hide knowledge gaps.

Also, when the attending physician admits what he does not know and models what he does to teach himself, this discourages students and residents from playing the "pretend to know" game.

Sometimes humor can play a role in discouraging game playing. Here I am reminded of the teacher who asks a student, "What is the true function of the spleen?" The student, thinking he is supposed to know, says "I forgot." You see, he thinks that forgetting is better than not knowing. Then the teacher replies, "What a shame. The one person in the world who knows, and he forgot!"

PROBLEM–BASED TEACHING

Medical students can achieve instructional **objectives** by receiving a set of patient problems rather than a series of topics. Presenting a series of topics is the more traditional approach and is called **subject–based teaching**. Teachers may feel (a) less confident that the problem–based approach will cover (or uncover!) all the important concepts, but (b) more confident that what is learned will be recalled and used when the students have to manage patients with those problems. In a review of the literature on problem solving in higher education (Whitman 1983) and in medical education (Whitman and Schwenk 1986), there is widespread support for the notions that students learn as much information in problem–based as in subject–based instruction, and that what is learned is more accurately remembered and used in the future.

Problem–based teaching can be combined with either **teacher–centered learning** or **student–centered learning**. When combined with teacher–centered learning, the instructor delivers a lecture, but uses cases rather than topics to organize the presentation. When combined with student–centered learning, the instructor leads a **group discussion** of cases.

While some teachers may feel that students can learn "something" from any case, case studies used in the problem–based approach should aim for a higher level of expectation. The cases should be chosen to define and interpret the instructional objectives and must motivate the students to learn. Therefore, the cases presented to students cannot be serendipitous, but rather must be a *conscious choice*.

For example, a subject–based approach to teaching "functional impairments of the elderly" might include five subtopics: (1) failure to ambulate, (2) falling, (3) failure to eat or drink adequately, (4) incontinence, and (5) intellectual impairment. However, if a teacher decided to use a problem–based approach, cases would have to be chosen that addressed all five impairments.

While it is important that cases address instructional objectives, it is also helpful for cases to be interesting. Interesting cases tend to be better learning tools because they are motivating for students and create a memorable experience to help trigger recall of information for future use. Thus, developing cases is a *creative process*.

Ruthanne Ramsey, Pharm. D., a creative case–developer and an associate of the Intermountain West

Geriatrics Education Center, recommends that the patient be given an interesting name. Rather than initials such as S.M., call the patient Sophie Malcowitz. Second, relate some unusual personal details about the patient. Perhaps the patient is the "oldest living diabetic in the United States" or " a Federal prisoner convicted of international forgery" or was "General MacArthur's personal secretary." Rather than just stating that an 82–year–old woman has a decubitus ulcer on the left buttock, describe the ulcer as "adjacent to a fantastic three–color tattoo of a parrot." Also, remember that bizarre things happen to real people. Maybe the suspicion of squamous cell lung cancer was first aroused after a chest radiograph ordered by an oral surgeon, who though the patient swallowed an instrument during a procedure (Ramsey and Whitman 1989).

No two teachers will write the same case and some teachers tend to incorporate more emotional elements such as humor or drama in the creation of cases. By making conscious choices and being as creative as possible, teachers can develop cases that meet course objectives and are memorable. In addition to choosing between the subject–based and the problem–based approach, teachers also have to decide who will be responsible for what is learned: the teacher or the student.

Some medical schools have made problem–based, student–centered learning the thrust of their curriculum (see **Harvard's New Pathway** and **The New Mexico Experiment**). But creative teachers can also make these changes in a traditional curriculum. For example, Dr. Thomas G. Hollinger at the University of Florida included a problem–based module in addition to the standard lectures in his embryology course. Eight or nine students were assigned to each group and were presented with clinical signs and symptoms of an unknown embryological problem.

The group had to decide what information to request, what approach to take, and what resources to use. Each student was required at least once to conduct a computerized literature search. Based on his observations and the student evaluations, Hollinger concluded that,

> The problem–based component encouraged students to think in terms of defining the questions they needed to ask, how to get answers to the questions they posed, how to assemble data and how to communicate this information to others (1989, p. 45).

PROBLEM SOLVING

Problem solving leads to a value for an unknown and usually encompasses both a strategy and elements of skill necessary to carry out that strategy. Its solution entails the best, but not necessarily the sole, answer. The importance of teaching problem solving in medicine was noted by the AAMC General Professional Education of the Physician report, *Physicians for the Twenty–First Century* (1984), which identified as essential to all physicians the ability to identify, formulate, and solve problems (see **GPEP Report**).

Research in this field supports the notion that most physicians follow similar problem solving steps and that effective problem solving depends upon the retrieval of relevant content from a well–organized store of long term memories (Elstein *et al.* 1978). Studies of medical problem solving suggest that instruction not be directed at the problem solving process, but rather at more specific behaviors that can be changed, such as knowledge acquisition and data gathering techniques (Neufield *et al.* 1981).

Every medical educator should read Ms. Christine H. McGuire's critique of the literature presented at the 1984

Conference on Research in Medical Education at the Annual Meeting of the Association of American Medical Colleges, in which she criticized both the medical community and the educational research community. With regard to the medical community, studies of clinical reasoning reveal that all too often physicians do not collect the data they need, do not pay attention to data they collect, and do not use their knowledge effectively in interpreting the data they do consider. With respect to the educational researchers, McGuire was critical of their methodology and tendency to overgeneralize. "In short, individuals in both communities are prone to human error, and performance in both must be improved" (1985, p. 594).

How can medical teachers help their students and residents learn to become better problem solvers? They will become better problem solvers when they are actively engaged in problem solving. Thus, the teacher's role is to involve the learners in the process by asking questions and letting the learners do most of the talking. Teachers should demonstrate good **problem solving attitudes** and avoid **problem solving biases.** The importance of role modeling cannot be over–emphasized. Negative role models, to be avoided, were identified by Dr. Lucien Israel, a French oncologist (1982):

1. The *unknowing* decision–maker works more on reflex than reflection, relying on an intuitive combination of what he knows and remembers.

2. The *ignorant* decision–maker doesn't know an answer and doesn't know he doesn't know it.

3. The *careless* decision–maker takes every risk, ending up with complications and treating them with catastrophic results.

4.   The *cautious* decision–maker sticks with the tried and true, laying blame on nature rather than conservative therapy.

5.   The *hurried* decision–maker rushes from one case to another, wanting our sympathy and help with the heavy cross he bears.

6.   The *unpredictable* decision–maker always has an opinion, but changes it constantly with the circumstances.

7.   The *depressed* decision–maker is tired and has lost faith, having invested a great deal, both intellectually and psychologically, in his self–image.

8.   The *temperamental* decision–maker roars when someone asks him a question and loses his temper if a patient wants a second opinion.

9.   The *inconsistent* decision–maker, according to his mood, will react differently to two identical situations.

10.   The *falsely systematic* decision–maker has formulated a few ideas which he applies no matter what the situation.

PROBLEM SOLVING ATTITUDES

Professor Donald Woods, who has designed a creative approach to teaching **problem solving** in the field of engineering at McMasters University, has identified ten attitudes which he thinks are essential to good problem solving. I presented this list at the 1988 Symposium of the Association of Pathology Chairmen (Prichard, Gardner, Jr., and Anderson 1989 and Whitman 1990) where participants confirmed its applicability to medical problem solving. To this list, I have added relevant quotations from the world of philosophy and literature:

1. Are you *careful*?
    "Education is turning things over in the mind."
    Robert Frost

2. Are you *attentive*?
    "Training means learning the rules. Experience means learning the exceptions." Anonymous

3. Are you *curious*?
    "Supposing is good, but finding out is better." Mark Twain

4. Are you *skeptical*?
    "There are four causes of ignorance—faith in authority, the power of custom, illusions of sense, and the proud delusion of ingrained wisdom." Roger Bacon

5. Are you *honest*?
    "There are four sorts of men: He who knows not and knows not; he is a fool—shun him. He who knows not and knows he knows not; he is simple—teach him. He who knows and knows not he knows; he is asleep—wake him. He who knows and knows he knows; he is wise—follow him." Robert Burton

6. Are you *objective*?
    "All human knowledge is but picking and culling. Because the false mixes with the true, it is no excuse for rejecting the mass." Victor Hugo

7. Are you *receptive*?
    "Some people will never learn anything, for this reason, because they understand everything too soon." Alexander Pope

8.   Are you *systematic*?
        "It is the duty of good education to arrive at wisdom by means of a definite order." St. Augustine

9.   Are you *decisive*?
        "To spend too much time in studies is sloth." Francis Bacon

10.   Are you *persistent*?
        "To question is to have the will to know." Martin Heidegger

PROBLEM SOLVING BIASES

Nothing is more dangerous than an idea when it is the only one we have.

Problem solving is an important skill for medical teachers to be good **role models**, especially when they teach. However, they may be subject to biases. In one study of surgeons, three potential biases were identified (Detmer, Fryback, and Gassner 1978). First, medical teachers could be insensitive to sample size. Although it is a statistical fact that there is greater variability with smaller sample sizes, on a question designed to test for this bias, twenty of thirty–eight surgeons gave answers inconsistent with sampling theory.

Second, some medical teachers practice "gambler's fallacy," *i.e.*, the belief that chance events are self–correcting. For example, ten heads in a row while flipping a coin does not make tails "due" on the eleventh toss. Yet, on a question designed to test for this phenomenon, one–third of the surgeons were influenced by this bias.

Finally, light of hindsight can be revealing, *i.e.*, the occurrence of events which seemed unpredictable in prospect may appear predictable in retrospect. To test for this bias, the surgeons were randomly assigned to three groups.

All groups were given a case description compatible with abdominal aortic aneurysm (AAA). Group #1 was informed that an AAA was found and resected. Group #2 was told that a tortuous aorta was noted on operation. Group #3 was given no additional information. All three groups were asked, "Based on the information available before the operation, what would you have estimated as the probability that this patient had a leaking AAA?" Detmer and colleagues found that outcome information had an obvious effect on their predictions.

Other types of problem solving errors have been classified. Kern and Doherty (1982) have described *pseudodiagnosticity*, that is, seeking data that will not be helpful. Voytovich *et al.* (1985) reported on *wrong synthesis* (making an unwarranted conclusion) and *inadequate synthesis* (not making a warranted conclusion). They also described *premature closure* and *anchoring*. Whereas premature closure hinders the search for additional data because the decision–maker thinks he is done, anchoring retards a response to new information because he feels secure in his diagnosis. Friedlander and Phillips (1984) found that experienced clinicians may be more susceptible to anchoring than medical students and residents, who are less willing to hold onto an earlier diagnosis in the face of conflicting data.

Clinical teachers should be alert to their own vulnerability to these problem solving biases as well as that of their medical students and residents so that commission of these errors can be a basis for discussion and learning. The right attitude of clinical teachers is a key element in promoting good problem solving (see **problem solving attitudes**).

PROFESSIONAL INTIMACY

Medical student and resident performance will be enhanced when their teachers are emotionally close without being necessarily personal friends—a delicately balanced relationship called "professional intimacy" (Whitman and Schwenk 1984). An analogous relationship exists between doctors and patients. On one hand, it is neither possible nor desirable for physicians to make every patient a close, personal friend. On the other hand, interaction is improved when physicians do not hide behind a facade.

Being professionally intimate with medical students and residents means *sharing your thoughts and values* in a manner that encourages them to share theirs with you and *demonstrating comfort* with learners of different abilities and backgrounds. Faculty who are professionally intimate often become positive **role models** for medical students and residents, *i.e.*, someone who does not *tell* others how to be but can *show* them and, by example, make being that way seem desirable and worthwhile.

When teachers are professionally intimate, the "psychological distance" between teachers and learners lessens so that medical students, residents, and faculty can teach each other and engage in a **conversation of medicine** in which all participants become learners.

QUESTIONING

Questioning is an important teaching **technique** because it establishes two–way communication. This is critical even in a **lecture.** For example, a question can be used at the start of a lecture to get audience members thinking about the subject, or mid–way into a lecture to provoke audience participation. Keep in mind that every question does not have a single, correct answer. Asking a question can be particularly effective when the question contains a sense of wonder. Lewis Thomas, Chancellor of the Memorial Sloan–Kettering Cancer Center, once commented that science is taught as if the facts were somehow superior to the facts in all the other scholarly disciplines. He called for more recognition that every field of science is incomplete (1982). The uncertainties of medicine were highlighted by Bursztajn et al., who describe a "probabilistic paradigm" of medicine in their thoughtful book, *Medical Choices, Medical Chances* (1981).

Questioning obviously is a key to effective **group discussion** leadership. It allows a leader to initiate discussion, encourage participation, and keep the discussion on track. Before a group discussion, it is helpful to formulate questions that are clear and succinct. During the discussion, avoid questions that are vague, complex, and wordy (McBeath and Lane 1977). Both closed and open–ended questions are recommended (Foley and Smilansky 1980). Closed questions include *memory* questions that ask for repetition of what has been learned, e.g., "Is 180 degrees a normal range of motion for a shoulder abduction?" and *convergent* questions that ask for recall and use of information, e.g., "How does the release of epinephrine into the blood change blood pressure?" Open–ended questions include *process* questions aimed at problem solving, e.g., "An experimental animal weighing 150g is given 1000mg of glucose and after two hours dies—what might be the cause of death?" and *evaluation* questions which ask students to take and defend a position, e.g., "What do you think has contributed most to the control of infectious disease?"

Closed and open–ended questions also can be used during hospital rounds. On geriatrics rounds, the attending physician could ask, "How is creatinine clearance estimated in geriatric patients?" (memory question). "Using the Cockcroft and Gault formula, what is this patient's creatinine clearance?" (convergent question). "If the projected creatinine clearance is less than twenty, how would you dose the digitalis?" (process question). "How useful is the Cockcroft and Gault formula in clinical application?" (evaluation question).

Clinicians tend to use all four types of questions when interviewing patients, whether they realize it or not. They use an interviewing style that I liken to playing the accordion: open–ended questions let the patient provide some direction, closed questions focus on an issue, and open–ended questions are used again to identify other issues. This process of using open–ended, closed, and open–ended questions again also works well in teaching (see **clinical teaching is like clinical care**). Whereas closed questions are helpful to determine whether the learner knows and understands information, open–ended questions help to stimulate thinking.

In a study of third–year medical students, Foster (1983) investigated the relationship between the cognitive level of teachers' questions and the level of the students' answers. She found that higher level questions elicited higher level answers. This may seem like common sense, hardly requiring educational research. However, her study revealed a more interesting finding: clinical teachers, perhaps because they particularly appreciate the responses of brighter students, may unwittingly direct more of their higher level questions to the better students. Creative teachers should consider challenging the thinking of all students rather than saving their most difficult questions for the students they believe are best prepared to answer.

Overall, a problem with higher education is that teachers talk too much. In typical classes, professors talk eighty percent of the time. Not only do they talk a great deal, but they take little time to ask questions and most of their questions ask for recall of facts. According to a study of classroom teaching conducted by Ellner and Barnes (1983), medical school teachers take more time than college teachers to ask questions (seven versus four percent), but ask fewer questions above the factual level (ten percent versus twenty percent). An additional problem is that teachers do not tolerate silence and give students little time to answer (see **wait times**).

The problems with questioning apply to clinical as well as classroom teaching. In a study of teacher–student interactions in a medical clerkship, Foley *et al.* used two gross indices of medical student involvement: ratio of teacher–to–student talk and level of student thinking required by the attending physician. After analysis of videotapes, they found that medical students by and large function as a passive audience. For example, on teaching rounds, medical students talked only four percent of the time whereas residents talked thirty–three percent and instructors sixty–two percent. Only seventeen percent of the talk was devoted to questions and eighty–one percent of the questions were low level. If teachers do most of the talking, we must question who is doing most of the learning!

RAIMI

Ralph A. Raimi, a professor of mathematics at the University of Rochester, sometimes finds himself teaching something that someone else has taught before him. Overlap also occurs in medical education and, like Raimi, you may have found it difficult to get the attention of learners (see **attention span**). You may want to adapt his introductory speech for such cases:

Many of you already know what I am about to tell you, but some of you do not. Those who do know—please be patient. You do not complain, when you attend a concert, that you have heard Beethoven's Seventh Symphony before, do you? Well, the Law of Cosines is just as lovely a monument to the human spirit.

You may complain if I give a bad performance, sure; but if I do it competently, this repetition of a thing of beauty should be a pleasure to you, even more than to those of your classmates who, not having your experience behind them, will have to strain their powers to follow me this first time around.

Raimi explains to fellow teachers that he then goes on to make the performance one of concert quality, but not entirely for the reasons advertised:

I know from experience, you see, that precious few of those students actually do understand the Law of Cosines. Many think so, having heard the words before, and would therefore mistakenly tune out my exposition, did I not first give them a self–respecting reason for listening.

RATING FORMS

The most common format for student evaluation of teachers (see **student ratings**) and for teacher evaluation of clinical student performance (see **student evaluation**) is the rating form (Whitman and Cockayne 1984). Basically, a rating form is an instrument that requires the observer to assign a numerical value to specific items. Ratings are subjective assessments made on an established scale. By collecting ratings from a representative sample of respondents, individual respondent biases presumably are cancelled out.

As you develop the items to be rated, please consider only important aspects of performance. Each item should contain only one thought, stated in a short, concise statement. With regard to the rating scale, a continuum of "excellent" to "poor" or a Likert scale of "strongly agree" to "strongly disagree" can be helpful. Then decide whether you prefer an odd–numbered scale which provides a neutral rating in the middle or an even–numbered scale that forces a positive or negative response. In any case, there should be no fewer than three and no more than seven positions on the scale, with an additional position for "not observed" or "do not know."

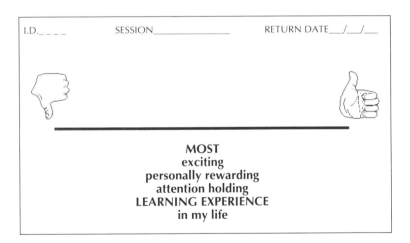

When I want a global rating for a workshop on teaching skills, I sometimes ask participants to think of their most exciting, personally rewarding, attention–holding, learning experience. Then I ask them to compare my workshop to *that* experience! They are provided a card with a line drawn between a thumbs–up and a thumbs–down icon. This is an

open–ended scale with no preset positions. They simply
mark the line where they think my workshop falls. If I want
a post–workshop follow up, perhaps three months later, I
provide self–addressed, stamped postcards. By asking for the
last four digits of their social security number, I can anony-
mously compare how individuals felt immediately after the
workshop to how they feel after they have had time to imple-
ment the skills taught at the workshop.

REMEMBERING

When a friend of Edmund Blair Bolles (1988) apolo-
gized for forgetting something, he quipped, "It's my 64K
memory." His **metaphor** was that the brain is a computer
chip. Because every computer has memory, discussions of
human memory often use words drawn from computer
terminology, including concepts like "storage" and "retrieval
of information." Actually, according to Bolles, people have
believed for several thousand years that remembering re-
trieves information stored somewhere in the brain. Even
before the invention of the computer, metaphors of memory
have used the concept of storage. For example, we speak of
carving memories in stone or preserving images on wax. We
file memories away. We retain facts in a steel trap. We say
that some people have photographic memories.

The traditional view of memory is that it consists of
three stages: (1) acquisition of new material, (2) storage of
the material in the brain, and (3) retrieval of the material
when it is needed. The conventional wisdom was that when
something could not be remembered, there was a problem
with one of these stages. When a student cannot remember
something, the teacher usually thinks the problem is in stage
three, *i.e.*, the student cannot retrieve what was taught.
Although it is convenient to describe memories as if they
were notes in filing cabinets or data banks in computers, the

fact is that these metaphors do not explain the way experiences are reflected in the brain.

Memory is not a tangible object, a note we make to ourselves and put away for future reference. Instead, every experience or encounter with our environment, including reading this page or listening to a lecture, modifies our nervous system. What we learn is a reflection of changes in the structure and connection of neurons in our brain. At the cellular level, experiences change the chemical activities of neurons, and at the anatomical level, these chemical changes lead to new interactions between neurons, producing new pathways which allow the brain to function in new ways.

However, the brain is more than a biochemical device in which memory is a passive response manipulated by objective factors such as the words on this page or the voice of a lecturer. The biochemical changes are not the same every time you read the same words or listen to the same lecture. John Stone, a cardiologist who teaches at Emory University Medical School, noted that, "Affection, rage, joy, argument and reconciliation, jealousy, every powerful emotion, can cause memory areas of our brains to light up like a multicolored PET scan" (1989, p. 60).

Thus, instead of the brain being like a computer, Bolles suggests that it is more like a piano and memory like the playing of a tune. Memory gives us new ways to perform. Desire, attention, and judgment all play a role in what we remember. Working backwards, we remember what we understand, we understand what we pay attention to, and we pay attention to what we want. When memory fails, the problem lies in one of those links in the chain.

John Russell, the art critic for *The New York Times*, wrote that, "No two human beings read the same book, watch the same play, sit through the same movie or look at the same paintings or sculptures. Different eyes and different ears are at work, and different expectations" (1989). Thus, when you deliver a lecture, lead a group discussion, or supervise medical students or residents in a hospital ward, what is learned and remembered is up to the learner. In a sense, there always is learning. The question is: "What do you want them to learn and what can you do to make that possible?"

RESIDENT EVALUATION

There are two types of resident evaluation. *Formative* evaluation is conducted while the process of teaching and learning occurs, and its purpose is to improve resident performance. In this sense, it is a type of **feedback.** *Summative* evaluation is conducted at the end of the **teaching–learning process**, and its purpose is to rate residents so that decisions can be made about their readiness to move to the next year or to graduate (Scriven 1967).

Comprehensive evaluation of residents recognizes four levels of resident performance (McLagan 1978):

1.   How motivated is the resident?

2.   How well is the resident handling his clinical responsibilities?

3.   How well is the resident achieving the goals and objectives of the program?

4.   How well is the resident applying what is being learned to clinical care?

The key to confidently evaluating those four levels of resident performance is to use multiple sources of data (Rutman 1980). Systematic evaluation of residents makes use of five data sources (Whitman 1983):

- observation by faculty using concurrent tools, such as checklists, critical incident forms, observation forms, and anecdotal records (see **clinical performance testing**), and retrospective tools, such as end–of–rotation **rating forms**, to assess levels 1 through 4;

- peer review by other residents (only if the environment discourages negative bias due to competition or positive bias due to cooperation) to assess levels 1 through 4;

- self–report by residents where they are asked to compare intended to actual performance to assess levels 1 through 4;

- standardized tests such as inservice examinations to assess level 3; and

- chart review by faculty to assess level 4.

RESIDENTS AS TEACHERS

Perhaps in no other aspect of medical education do I feel as personally invested as I do in teaching residents to teach. I usually begin "Residents as Teachers" workshops by asking them why they think their residency director asked me to meet with them. Almost always, they cite their responsibilities for teaching other residents and medical students. Sometimes they respond that they learn when they teach and, perhaps, if they taught more effectively, they would learn more. This response corresponds to my strong sense that residents should be taught how to teach. Dr. Thomas L. Schwenk and I, in our handbook for resident teachers, address this issue on page one:

> Intuitively, doesn't it make sense that, in the
> act of organizing, preparing, and presenting
> materials to others, you learn a lot in the

process? By your being a better teacher for
others, we are convinced that you will be the
best teacher for yourself (1984).

Kent J. Sheets, a Ph.D. educator who works with Tom
Schwenk at the University of Michigan, reviewed the literature on the resident's teaching role. He found that many
residents would like to be better teachers, but lack the time
to complete faculty development training traditionally offered to faculty. He concluded that a minimalist approach
using a two or three hour workshop may be optimal, with
one–to–one consultation and additional group sessions
provided at the request of interested residents (1988). As a
resource for anyone planning a program to teach residents to
teach, a comprehensive guide is provided by Janine Edwards,
Ph.D. and Robert Marier, M.D., editors of *Resident Teaching:
Rules, Techniques, and Programs* (1988).

Personal experience confirms their recommendation
that residency directors play a key role in influencing the
role of the resident as a teacher. For instance, in 1985 I was
asked to join a surgery team for one week to observe the
chief resident's teaching and give him feedback. From Mon-
day through Thursday, I joined the team in its daily activities: rounding at 6:30 a.m., scrubbing at 8:00 a.m., making
rounds in the afternoon, *etc.* Most of the discussion during
rounds centered on patient management and few team
members participated. On Friday, I asked the team if I could
audiotape rounds so that I could make a transcript. The chief
resident replied, "Sure, but I guess I'll have to teach today!"
And he did! And at 8:00 a.m. we were scrubbing in the O.R.
on time. What "**teaching**" could have occurred and why did
it not make rounds take longer?

Teaching occurred during surgery rounds not with
mini–lectures, but with helpful interactions. For example,
while leaving a post–surgical patient's room, the chief

resident asked a fourth–year medical student, "By the way, was that person a good candidate for vascular surgery?" Before seeing a new patient on the service, the chief resident asked an intern, "What type of tumor is most apt to cause shoulder pain in this 60–year–old man?" Later, when a resident presented the case of a 27–year–old woman admitted with a chief complaint of abdominal pain, the chief resident asked other team members what gynecologic history they wanted to hear (see **questioning**).

From this experience, I learned that this chief resident could teach more effectively when he thought it was important to do so. For that reason I particularly appreciate the recommendation of Dr. Fred J. Schiffman, who teaches internal medicine at Brown University: residency directors should communicate the importance of resident teaching by working with residents to nurture their skills. In addition, he recommends an evaluation system to assess the success of residents as teachers (1986). The importance of **feedback** to residents was highlighted for me when I asked residents to evaluate themselves and medical students and faculty to evaluate these same residents. The residents thought they were not good teachers, whereas the students thought they were fair to good and the faculty thought they were good to excellent. When I showed these results to the residents, they were delighted that they were more successful than they had originally thought.

ROLE MODEL

So what makes a good teacher? Knowledge is necessary, but hardly sufficient. Every bit as important is how you impart information. How effectively you communicate is more important than how much you know; if you cannot get ideas across, you will not be an effective teacher and thus cannot be an effective physician. The ability to motivate and stimulate is

*critical to a successful teacher...because most effective teaching
is by example. Teachers are role models for their students,
demonstrating knowledge, clinical acumen, and other qualities
of a good physician (Miller 1990).*

Role modeling, or teaching by example, is intrinsic to
the process of teaching. Medical teachers are, whether they
realize it or not, role models for medical students and residents. Basic science teachers serve as role models by demonstrating the scientific method, including hypothesis testing.
Clinical teachers serve as role models by demonstrating
medical **problem solving** and bedside manners. Both basic
science and clinical teachers role model by conveying
enthusiasm for their work.

Teachers identified by graduating medical students as
enthusiastic were enlisted by the University of Chicago
Pritzker School of Medicine to interview patients in front of a
class of second–year medical students and, afterwards, to
discuss these interviews with the students. Siegler *et al.*
(1977) reported that, based on student questionnaires, this
simple change in the curriculum had a positive effect on
student attitudes (see **attitudinal change**) and that "the use
of such role models should be considered as a means of
improving the teaching of the doctor–patient relationship
and of improving students' attitudes about the importance of
interpersonal skills" (p. 937).

In order to promote role modeling, the Indiana
University School of Medicine convened a conference for
approximately 100 faculty members, community physicians,
residents, and medical students, at which they concluded
that role modeling was essential to instilling within students
the desire to become lifelong learners (Ficklin *et al.* 1988).

Although the Indiana participants identified both
positive and negative aspects of role modeling, when some

educators use the term "role model" they assume a positive influence. However, role models can be positive or negative (see **teacher abuse**) In order to become a positive role model, medical teachers should consider four areas of professional behavior (Whitman and Schwenk 1984).

1. *Be capable.* You can teach medical students and residents to become competent clinicians by providing excellent medical care, being organized in your patient care and your teaching, being well–read in your field, and demonstrating how you value the development of your own abilities.

2. *Be sensitive.* You can teach medical students and residents to be sensitive by being sensitive to them as well as to your patients. Be empathic to the anxieties of being a medical learner, be patient with their efforts to learn, and be compassionate about their failures and gentle in recognizing their inadequacies. By treating your students and residents as you would like them to treat their patients, you will encourage proper approaches to patient care.

3. *Be enthusiastic.* When you demonstrate interest in your patients, medical students and residents become interested, as well. In addition, by being accessible to medical students and residents, concerned with their problems and needs and energetic in your approach to them, you will promote productive learning as well as good patient care. Most studies of teaching identify the importance of enthusiasm.

4. *Be yourself.* There is no single "good" personality type in Medicine. But, all positive role models are honest about how they deal with the uncertainties, difficulties, and ambiguities of medical practice.

In addition to considering these four areas of professional behavior, Irby (1986) suggests that to be an *intentional*
role model, medical teachers should articulate the mental
processes that led to the successful completion of a diagnosis
or clinical procedure. By demonstrating a skill *and* labelling
its important aspects, students and residents will be better
enabled to imitate it.

Related to the concept of role modeling is the notion
that medical teachers should establish **professional
intimacy**, *i.e.*, in a manner analogous to doctor–patient
relationships, teachers should be close to medical students
and residents without necessarily becoming personal friends.
By being professionally intimate with all medical students
and residents, a medical teacher will become a role model for
some. By being a role model for some medical students and
residents, a medical teacher may become a **mentor** for a few.

ROLE PLAYING

Role playing is a **technique** in which people tempo-
rarily adopt a specified role and try to behave in ways characteristic of that person in a specific situation. Role plays can
be used in a **lecture** to break up the "I talk, you listen" mode
of communication or in a small group to provide a focus for
group discussion.

For example, in the middle of a one–hour lecture on
taking adolescent histories, a pediatric teacher asked a resident to play the role of an adolescent sent for an assessment
because he had been "acting out" in school. Another resident
was asked to play the role of the examining physician. This
role play provided the lecturer with an opportunity later in
the lecture to highlight the importance of confidentiality to
the adolescent patient, the need to be non–judgmental, and

the relevance of developmental staging in assessing adolescents.

When using this technique, be as specific as possible in assigning the roles to be played and describing the situations in which the participants should play the role. Avoid interruption of the players and, when the role play is over, give the players and the observers an opportunity to comment on the experience.

Role playing is particularly appropriate when the instructional **objectives** include **attitudinal change** such as enhancing **humanistic behavior**. Rather than "telling students how to be" it is more effective to let them "discover how to be."

SHARKS

Voltaire Cousteau, the nom de plume of Richard J. Johns, has developed six rules to help medical students and residents swim with sharks. He points out that although nobody wants to swim with sharks and it is not an enjoyable sport, some people find themselves in shark–infested waters. Swimming with sharks is like other sports in that it cannot be learned by books alone. It is necessary to practice, and his rules are intended to help novices survive while becoming expert through practice:

1. Do not bleed.

2. Get out of the water if someone else is bleeding.

3. Assume unidentified fish are sharks.

4.   Counter any aggression promptly.

5.   Use anticipatory retaliation.

6.   Disorganize an organized attack.

       In all good conscience, I recommend only rules one, two, and three to medical students and residents. In any case, learning (and surviving) to swim with sharks is essential to using feedback (see **feedback, getting**).

SIMULATION

       One of the most creative **techniques** to teach or evaluate medical students and residents is the simulation. Essentially, a simulation places an individual in a setting that imitates reality. For example, it may be helpful to allow medical students or residents to practice a psychomotor **skill** on **teaching models** before performing that procedure on a patient. Photographs and audio–recordings can be used to reproduce diagnostic signs. Paper and pencil or computer-ized patient management problems can provide practice in clinical **problem solving**.

       A particularly innovative use of simulation is to mimic doctor–patient interactions. In the Department of Family and Community Medicine at the University of Toronto, each resident in a small group session returns a simulated message from an answering service to call a patient. The resident uses a speaker telephone so that the instructor and other residents can hear both sides of the conversation when the resident talks to the simulated patient (a physician trained in Psychiatry and Pediatrics). After the call is completed, the group discusses the encounter (Dunn, Norton, and Dunn 1987).

       Before using any of these types of simulations, it is helpful to first give an overview of its purpose. Then, when the activity is over, it is important to debrief and discuss the experience. The advantage of the simulation technique is that it can allow medical students and residents to anticipate real–life problems in a safe setting. Simulations both stimulate and reinforce learning. While a simulation can be as simple as audio–recordings of heart sounds, it can be as complex as "Harvey," a life–size manikin capable of simulating the bedside findings for a variety of cardiovascular conditions (Gordon 1974).

An innovative simulation was used to teach the psychomotor skill of central venous access. In this simulation, developed by surgery resident John D. S. Reid (1988), postautopsy cadaver specimens were prepared to produce a realistic model for central venous access. By removing abdominal and chest viscera, he provided good exposure to the subclavian and femoral arteries and veins. In each specimen, Dr. Reid used a balloon catheter thrombectomy to remove arterial and venous residual clots. Cannulae were attached to both artery and vein, which were perfused with red and blue food coloring. Finally, flow was instituted in the arterial circulation by distal arteriotomy. During femoral vein cannulation, distal arterial run–off facilitated generation of a simulated femoral pulse by pulsed compressions of the arterial solution bags. This simulated pulse served as a landmark that could be used to locate the adjacent vein during the performance of intravenous access. In subclavian access, static venous distension with blue solution was obtained by backfilling the venous circulation. This procedure allowed the filled vein to be located during the performance of the percutaneous central vein access.

Using eleven cadavers, three medical students performed a total of thirteen central venous access procedures, using six subclavian and seven femoral vein sites. When the subclavian or femoral artery was mistakenly entered, this error was immediately apparent from the red solution in the aspirating syringe. Similarly, when the parietal apical pleura was inadvertently transgressed during subclavian vein insertion, air bubbles in the aspirating syringe were noted. Thus, the model of central venous access accurately mimicked the real–life performance of this procedure, thereby providing students with feedback on their success or failure.

According to a study of emergency femoral vein access, residents experienced an 11 percent failure rate with 14 percent requiring two attempts. The researchers noted that resident performance improved with practice (Swanson *et al* 1984.). Wouldn't it be better for all concerned to first provide practice with realistic simulations?

The ability to learn from mistakes without harming the patient also was made possible by a medical simulation developed by Dr. Richard Robb, director of Biotechnology Computer Resources at the Mayo Clinic. His program, *Analyze*, was nominated as a finalist in the Medicine and Health Care category for the 1990 Computerworld Smithsonian Awards. With this program, doctors can perform practice surgery on a computer workstation using a patient's X–ray images before going into real surgery (Harrington 1990).

SKILLS

See one. Do one. Teach one.

Dr. Mark A. Rockoff, as a third–year medical student at the Johns Hopkins University School of Medicine, recalled hearing during his medical school admission interviews that, "The way to learn here is to see one, do one, teach one." A problem he encountered as a medical student was that occasionally he did not get to see one before he had to do one (1973).

For medical students, life is full of opportunities to show off their ignorance. This often occurs when the instructional **objectives** are psychomotor. In describing how she learned to draw arterial blood, Dr. Perri Klass (1987) experienced a variation of the traditional surgical dictum: *See three. Try four. Miss them all.* Similarly, in learning how to perform a lumbar puncture, Dr. Melvin Konner (1987) followed another variation: *See one. Screw one. Do one.*

The problem a medical teacher may have in trying to "manage (their) ignorance into competence" (Konner) is that the instructor is too competent! He may know a procedure or skill so well that he is no longer conscious of the step–by–step process behind successful completion of the task. Therefore, he cannot communicate to the medical student what it takes to do the procedure or perform the skill. This problem of over–competence was first identified in the field of industrial training:

> They know their jobs so well that they no longer have to think about what they are doing. They have arrived at a point where they can perform a given task *unconsciously*. That is they are competent, but are *unconsciously competent*, and that's what makes them poor instructors. They are no longer conscious of the step–by–step process behind successful completion of the task. Therefore, they cannot communicate properly to a trainee— to an individual who is *consciously incompetent*—about what it takes to do this job (*Personnel Journal* 1974).

The solution to this problem is for teachers to recognize when the learner is unconsciously incompetent, with a need first to learn what it is that he cannot do. When the learner is consciously incompetent, *i.e.*, he cannot do something, but at least knows what it is he cannot do, then there is a need to help the learner become consciously competent, *i.e.*, perform the skill in a step–by–step format. This requires the unconsciously competent teacher to recall the steps that may now be performed automatically.

The need to join the learner at his level is evident when an eight–year old teaches another eight–year old how to play chess. Within ten minutes, they are playing a game that I would be willing to call "chess." The teacher knows the right language to use ("The horse moves this way") and the learner never doubts his ability to learn how to play the game. But, watch a chess master teach a novice how to play! The expert knows far too much and soon is discussing openings, middle games, and end games in too much detail. The beginner becomes far too confused and intimidated to master such a complicated game.

SLIDES

Two ophthalmology teachers wish things could be different:

> How exciting it would be, we thought as we attended a recent medical meeting, if a nondistracting audiovisual technique could be developed, one which did not overload the listener each 15 seconds with more material than could be observed. How rewarding it would be to be able to concentrate one's attention on a few important points made visually on a clearly discriminated slide, well–coordinated with the speaker's words (Kramer and Schwartz 1986, p.657)!

The fact that eye doctors made these comments is particularly appropriate because of the major abuse of slides:

projecting tables and graphs produced in enough detail for journals, but unsuitable for slides. If there is information in a table or graph, it should be abstracted and simplified for slides. A good rule of thumb is that audience members will not read more than thirty–five words on a slide. Ten to twelve words are recommended and the lettering should be at least $^1/_{15}$ of the height of the working area. Instead of having to apologize for bad slides, delete them (see **Kroenke's Rules**).

One medical educator borrows advice from the world of advertising, recommending that, if a slide is not under-stood in four seconds, it is a bad slide. Also, "You cannot bore people into buying." Do not use only word slides. Use pictures when appropriate to convey your ideas. (Evans 1978). Finally, do not project slides in a completely dark room. If there are no artificial light dimmers or natural light that can be let in with shades or curtains, do not use slides. Let's face it, medical teachers often are speaking to sleep–deprived audiences. What happens when the lights go off?

STRESS

Stress is our response to situations we perceive as unpleasant. Hans Selye, the so–called "father of stress," observed in 1936 that the effect of a chemical extract on rats had the same effects on the control group injected with a placebo: peptic ulcers, atrophy of immune system tissues, and enlargement of the adrenal glands. He concluded that the rats had a generalized response to the unpleasantness of the injections *per se*. He borrowed the word, *stress*, from engineering to describe the body's nonspecific response to an insult or threat.

Selye described this stress reaction as the General Adaptation Syndrome. First, there is an alarm reaction.

Second, there is resistance. Third, there is exhaustion. Today this is known as the "fight or flight" syndrome. When we perceive a physical threat, there is a chain of internal events that give us the resources to attack or run away. The problem today is that psychological threats evoke the same set of physiological responses which, in the long run, may compromise a person's physical health, particularly if the stress response is chronic.

Of course, to some extent, stress is helpful even in the face of psychological challenges. Without stress, there is entropy. Without stress, medical students and residents would learn little. However, lack of stress is not a problem in medical schools and residency programs. Our problem is too much stress, *i.e.*, distress, that leads to less learning (see **continuing medical education**). The analogy to explain this phenomenon is that of weight lifting. Strength will not be increased if the weights are too light. On the other hand, if the weights are too heavy, one risks injury. This relationship between stress and learning was identified as early as 1908 by Yerkes and Dodson and several supporting studies have been reviewed by Hockey (1979).

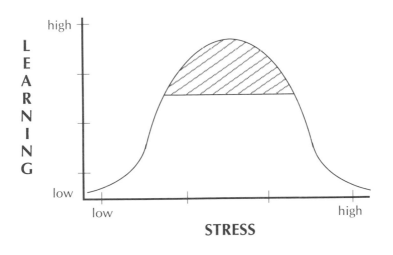

In teaching medical students and residents, it is important to note that not everyone is stressed by the same event. When stressed, everyone does not generate the same physiological response. In a study of dominant and subordinate baboons, Sapolsky (1990) found that subordinate baboons, whose social life is more stressful than dominant baboons, trigger more cortisol which, in turn, produces lower levels of circulating HDL cholesterol, the so–called "good" cholesterol. The lowest cortisol levels (and higher HDL levels) were found in baboons who could best differentiate between the neutral and threatening actions of rivals. This raises the issue of stress inoculation developed by Meichenbaum (1974) who suggested that humans can be prepared for stress by differentiating between situations that require response and those which do not and rehearsing for situations that are stressful.

You may wonder if research on free–ranging baboons in Kenya is relevant to a medical school or teaching hospital. However, Sapolsky's baboons provide a good model. These animals have abundant food supplies and few predators. With the luxury of plentiful resources and free time, these animals can devote themselves to distressing one another and, as described by Sapolsky, they "occupy a social landscape of Machiavellian dimensions" (see **pimping** and **sharks**).

What stresses most medical students and residents? A major stressor for first–year medical students is the amount and complexity of material to be learned. Students feel academic pressure because nearly all classmates are used to being above average (Gaensbauer and Mizner 1980). Fatigue is often cited as a stressor in the second year, and many medical researchers describe a hypochondriacal phenomenon as students imagine they have the diseases they are studying (Bojar 1971). In the third year, as medical students begin clinical rotations, they are low on the totem pole and begin to cope with issues such as death and dying. Fourth–year medical students deal with the stresses of residency selection and, in the first year of the residency, begin a process of overwork and sleep deprivation (Whitman, Spendlove, and Clark 1984). According to the National Institute of Workers Compensation, there are only four jobs in the United States more stressful than being a medical intern: air traffic controller, coal miner, police officer, and inner city high school teacher.

What can teachers do to help medical students and residents learn to cope with stress so that there is optimal learning? The key lies in **professional intimacy**, *i.e.*, the process of being emotionally close to them without necessarily being a social friend. How faculty interact with medical students and residents will have a major impact on learning (Whitman, Spendlove, and Clark 1986). A number of prominent people (including Paul Berg, a Nobel Prize winner in Chemistry; Beverly Sills, former opera star and manager of the New York City Opera; Kenneth Clark, noted psychologist and Civil Rights advocate) who were asked to recall teachers who had influenced them said, "Expectations. Respect. Understanding. Opening windows. These, rather than specific areas, are the characteristics that are repeated over and over" (Hechinger 1980b).

Surely, when you were a medical student or resident, there were **mentors** who helped you learn how to cope with the stresses of medical training by being themselves and being available. Creative teaching depends upon **role modeling**. While you cannot *tell* someone else how to be, you can *show* them and, by example, make being that way seem desirable and worthwhile.

STUDENT ABUSE

In 1982 (Silver) and again in 1984 (Rosenberg and Silver), the term "abuse" was used to draw the parallel between medical students and battered children. Is this highly charged term appropriate to describe the educational experiences of medical students? A major problem involves the definition and understanding of the word "abuse." Abuse is a subjective experience and can only be known and described by the subject (Baldwin *et al.* 1988).

In a study to describe the subjective experiences of medical students at one medical school, a questionnaire was administered at a student get–together. The questionnaire was completed by most of the students present, representing 42 percent of the junior and senior classes:

1.   With regard to *verbal* abuse, 19 percent of the students cited basic scientists, 26 percent attending physicians, and 34 percent residents.

2.   With regard to *physical* abuse, 2 percent of the students cited basic scientists, 4 percent attending physicians, and 9 percent residents.

3.   With regard to *sexual* abuse, 5 percent of the students cited basic scientists, 8 percent attending physicians, and 14 percent residents.

These responses raise a number of questions. Are basic scientists more benign or, since respondents were juniors and seniors, have past abuses been forgotten? If there is less abuse by basic scientists, is this due to less opportunity (less one–to–one contact)? Are residents more malicious than attending physicians or do they spend more time with students?

Finally, if it were possible to identify teachers who abuse students (anonymous self–report?), I would like to know their characteristics and whether they were abused as students (see **teacher abuse**).

STUDENT–CENTERED LEARNING

Whereas teachers determine what is to be learned in the **teacher–centered** classroom, students make these decisions in the student–centered classroom. In student–centered learning, the teacher recognizes the value of interpersonal interaction as the prime teaching modality and views the students as responsible for their own learning.

The teacher plays a facilitative role in student–centered learning. To begin with, teachers listen and encourage students to listen to each other. They observe. Does anyone have anything to say? Is there agreement or disagreement? Are students confused and in need of clarification? Are they bored and ready to move on? By paying attention to what is said and not said, the teacher gains a sense of student needs. In the student–centered classroom, teachers tolerate silence. They give students time to ask and answer questions. Teachers post important points on the board. They help keep track of the discussion and encourage students to participate.

As an example of this approach, the Department of Pathology at the Robert Wood Johnson Medical School in Piscataway, New Jersey, adopted a major change in their sophomore pathology course in which lectures were replaced with small–group discussions. Raskova and colleagues reported that the students' adjustment seemed to come gradually, with most students developing new learning habits and self–confidence by the end of the course (1988).

Student–centered learning can be combined with **subject–based** or **problem–based teaching**. With subject–based teaching, the instructor could ask students to discuss functional impairments of the elderly. For each impairment, for example, failure to ambulate, the teacher could ask, "What are its causes?" The group could brainstorm to generate a differential diagnosis explaining failure to ambulate and, with contributions from each group member, develop a systematic approach that no single student could generate alone. The group could then identify some questions worth investigating prior to the next session. Student–centered learning can also be combined with problem–based teaching. Instead of discussing five functional impairments of the elderly, the group could discuss cases chosen by the teacher which include these impairments.

In either approach, subject–based or problem–based, the teacher's role in student–centered learning is to (1) uncover what the students know and do not know and (2) guide them to the resources that will help them learn what they do not know. What students do not know is used as a stimulus for self–study and for future group discussion.

In a course for first–year medical students at the Medical College of Ohio, a problem–based, student–centered approach was used to correlate biochemistry and physiology with clinical applications. At first, the course was problem–based but teacher–centered. Each session began with the introduction of a patient by a faculty member, followed by student questioning of the patient and the faculty member. Then, faculty presented a series of short lectures on related topics. To broaden student responsibility, a more student–centered approach was adopted which required students to lead these sessions, including topic–related discussions following the patient interviews. Students assigned to lead these sessions met in advance with faculty to discuss the cases to be presented and to prepare their own essays on related topics. The students took responsibility for the basic science review and divided the review material between themselves. As students took more responsibility for these sessions, the faculty assumed the role of consultants. The evaluations of these changes support the notion that students can use their abilities to be both teachers (see **peer teaching**) and students in the application of basic science knowledge to the understanding of human disease (Saffran and Yeasting 1985).

A question asked by K. Patricia Cross, a noted educator, is "What can teachers do to cause learning?" She identified (1) actively involving students in the learning task, (2) giving students an opportunity to practice what you want them to learn, and (3) setting high, but attainable goals (1987). The problem–based, student–centered approach enables us to realize all three recommendations. Because it is student–centered, it provides active involvement; because it is problem–based, it gives students a chance to do what we want them to do (diagnose and treat patients); and because the teacher expects the students to find the answers, it sets high expectations.

STUDENT CONCENTRATION

Two British medical educators, Stuart and Rutherford, studied the concentration of medical students in **lectures** and found that it rose to a maximum in ten to fifteen minutes and then fell steadily until the end of the lecture. They hypothesized that the progressive fall in concentration during the second half of lectures may reflect:

1.   saturation of the audience with factual data;

2.   partial exhaustion of the teacher and students;

3.   student boredom; or

4.   the lack of variety in the teaching method.

In this study, which included twelve teachers, they found

that variations in student concentration were fairly uniform for each lecturer, and that some lecturers obtained a consistently higher level of concentration and were able to hold a longer **attention span.** These findings are consistent with my own observations. However, I found rather shortsighted their conclusion that, "The reasons for this are complex and require further study" (1978, p. 515). I think the reasons are simple and need no further study.

Some lecturers are able to maintain student attention because they address the relatively passive role of learners in the lecture method. They use **techniques** to attract and maintain attention. They break up the "I talk—You listen" relationship. They stimulate students to think, so that when minds inevitably wander, at least they are wandering on the subject!

I can guarantee one way to diminish student concentration: if your **slides** are dull, inaccurate, badly–made, and illegible students will either go to sleep or walk out (Evans 1978).

STUDENT EVALUATION

Imbedded in the word *evaluation* is the word *value*. When we evaluate, we make a judgment about the worth of something or someone. At its simplest, evaluation leads to a settled opinion that something is the case. Evaluation of students seeks to answer the question, "Is this individual competent?" The obvious prior question must be, "What is competence?"

According to the Clinical Evaluation Project, sponsored by the Association of American Medical Colleges (1983), faculty spend too much time worrying about the instruments and methods of evaluation. While good instruments and methods are important, I agree that more emphasis should be placed on *doing* the evaluation. For example, in looking at fund of knowledge and technical skills, faculty should focus more on what is to be assessed and defining their expectations of students than on developing **rating forms**. Then they should make subjective evaluations of students, using their best clinical judgment, to identify categories of students.

1.   For students who are viewed as *superior*, the task of evaluating is to document student performance so that good performance is reinforced and rewarded.

2.   For students who are viewed as *failing*, the task of evaluating is to document student weaknesses and to specify needed improvements (see **double o sevens**).

3.   For students who are viewed as *adequate*, the task of evaluating is to look more closely so that faculty can identify whether a student is in this category because (a) he really is average, (b) no one really knows him, or (c) he really is failing, but no one wants to say so.

In order to judge whether students are superior, failing, or adequate, it is important that clinical performance be measured on a regular basis with checklists, critical incident forms, observation logs, and anecdotal records (see **clinical performance testing**). When it is necessary to supplement the testing of clinical performance there are a variety of methods available to standardize evaluation. For example, non–physician patient instructors can be trained to evaluate student performance (Stillman *et al.* 1980). Simulated cases (paper and pencil or computerized) can be administered to assess problem solving skills. The Objective Structured Clinical Evaluation (OSCE) consists of a series of stations at which each student must perform a clinical skill before going on to the next station (Petrusa 1987).

STUDENT RATINGS

Some faculty are concerned that student ratings of their teaching are nothing more than popularity contests with warm, friendly, humorous, easy–grading instructors emerging as the winners. The fact is that the reliability and validity of student ratings in higher education have been studied to death. Here are some representative findings:

> A review of empirical studies indicates that students' ratings can provide reliable and valid information on the quality of courses and instruction…. Research findings suggest that the criteria used by students in their ratings of instructors had much more to do with the quality of the presentation of the material than the entertainment value of the course *per se* (Costin, Greenough, and Menges).

> A review of recent research concerned with student ratings of teaching indicates that such evaluations are not significantly influenced by background variables, and are valid, reliable, stable, generalizable, and useful (Overall and Marsh).

> Many studies address the concern that most student ratings are nothing more than a popularity contest…. In rating their instructors, students discriminate among various aspects of teaching ability. If a teacher tells great jokes and has students in the palm of his or her hand in the classroom, he or she will receive high ratings in humor and classroom manner, but these ratings do not influence students' assessments of other teaching skills (Aleamoni).

Teaching can be seen as a performing art. A distinctive style of presentation, ability to dramatize portions of a lecture, and displays of energy and enthusiasm arouse student interest, and, as such are desirable teacher traits...(but) it is important to remember that the highest student ratings are garnered by 'substance' teachers, not merely 'entertainers' (Seldin).

A test is valid if it measures what it is supposed to measure, so it is more meaningful to talk about the validity of inferences based on results obtained from a test than about the validity of the test *per se*. In other words, student evaluation of teaching is valid if we make correct inferences from it. What inferences can we make about teachers from student ratings? What students can tell us, that no one else can, is how *they experienced the instruction*. Clearly, while the goal is for them to learn a lot, we also want them to like what they learned. Motivation is a key element of learning because people remember what they understand, understand what they pay attention to, and pay attention to what they want to!

To faculty who still doubt the reliability and validity of student ratings, I would ask whether their evaluation of students can stand up to objective criteria. How much evidence is there that faculty evaluation of medical students and residents is not influenced by irrelevant traits such as being attentive and polite? How do faculty know that their so–called objective tests measure what they are supposed to measure? In a workshop I conducted for Pathology faculty on constructing multiple choice tests, they scored 50% on a test I put together using their own sophomore test items. My point is that if the tables were turned, and faculty evaluation of students were questioned, there would be less evidence to support them than is available to support student evaluation of their teachers.

Of course, student ratings are not equal to **teacher evaluation.** They are only one component. Other components include colleague ratings and student achievement results. It is only by looking at multiple data sources that we can make substantive statements about the overall performance of teachers.

STUDENT TESTS

There is only twenty minutes. You can't write much in twenty minutes, but you can cross out a great deal. (helpful advice by proctor to students at Oxford, as told by Sir Kenneth Clark)

Although the National Board of Medical Examiners provides an important function in standardizing medical student testing, it is still important for teachers to construct their own tests. Scarvia Anderson, a former vice president of the Educational Testing Service, once commented that teacher–made tests, more than any other educational device, tell students what the purpose of instruction is and what can be expected of them (1977). Standardized tests, such as those constructed by the Educational Testing Service and the National Board of Medical Examiners, are certainly important. However, the tests that teachers make themselves should not be subordinated and deserve our attention.

Constructing tests is one of the most significant aspects of the teaching–learning process and, as pointed out by two testing specialists at Kansas State University, Richard Owens and Victoria Clegg, is one of the most frustrating because teachers have had no or little training in writing tests (1983). Also, it takes time to write good tests. Medical school faculty may say that they do not have time. Whenever we do not take the time to do something as well as we could do it, we have made a choice and we must accept the consequences. When faculty choose not to take the time to properly construct their own tests, the consequences are not life–threatening and are even not job–threatening. Nevertheless, I would like to be persuasive that tests reflect a medical school's professional standards and influence the relationship of its students to its teachers. Tests that are well–made demonstrate to students that the teachers are interested in the teaching–learning process. In many ways, tests reflect a teacher's standards. A sloppy test, poorly written, lacking clear directions, containing factual as well as grammatical mistakes, may say as much about the overall performance of a teacher as a sloppy lecture, poorly presented, lacking clear objectives.

In addition to reflecting negatively on a teacher, deservedly so, a poorly constructed test can reflect poorly on a medical student, undeservedly so! If a test is badly designed, a competent student may underperform and score close to a student with poor mastery. In this case, we would say that inferences made about student mastery from this test are invalid.

Writing good tests is primarily important to assess student mastery of content. But, preparing good tests can also help faculty gain a perspective on what they are teaching. Many faculty already recognize that they learn from teaching and have shared the experience of the British physicist, Ernest Rutherford, who believed that he had not completed a scientific discovery until he was able to translate it into readily understandable language (Lowman 1984). In a similar vein, an English professor was once asked if he understood T.S. Eliot's *Four Quartets*. He scratched his head and replied, "I don't know. I never tried to write an exam on it."

Faculty who wish to construct a good test item should follow a six–step process:

First, teachers should determine what learning **objectives** are to be measured. Of course, this assumes that learning objectives have been developed in the first place. Properly developed learning objectives represent what students should know and do in each content area or unit of a course and, taken together, describe the students' achievement of the overall course goals.

Second, teachers should identify the level of learning necessary for students to carry out each objective. Let's consider a course unit on HIV infection and AIDS. The lowest level cognitive objective is *basic knowledge* which requires simple recall of material. For example, "Identify five high risk behaviors for HIV infection." A higher level objective requiring *comprehension* would be for students to explain why these behaviors are high risk. *Application* refers to the ability to use the learned material in new ways or new situations. For example, given a patient's history, can the student assess that person's risk for HIV infection?

Analysis, synthesis, and evaluation reflect higher levels of student learning and require higher levels of performance. Analysis refers to the ability to break down material into its parts so that its organizational structure can be understood. For example, "The student should be able to compare the psycho–social aspects of AIDS to other chronic diseases." Synthesis refers to the ability to put the parts together in a new way. For example, "The student should be able to relate ways in which a patient's developmental age might affect adjustment to AIDS." Evaluation, the highest level of cognitive learning, is concerned with the ability to make judgments. For example, "The student should be able to critique the University Hospital's AIDS policies and procedures for the testing of staff and recommend improvements."

	Matching	True/False	Short Answer	Problem Solving	Multiple Choice	Essay
Evaluation						●
Synthesis			●	●	●	●
Analysis			●	●	●	●
Application			●	●	●	
Comprehension	●	●	●	●		
Knowledge	●	●	●			

Third, faculty should match the test to the objectives, not the objectives to the test. Each type of test item has a place in testing students. Matching items, true–false items, and short answer items are good for testing basic knowledge, but are inappropriate for higher level objectives. Since students can answer four matching questions or three true–false questions in a minute, their advantage is that faculty can measure more objectives in the same amount of time. Conversely, because students may be able to answer only one or two short answer questions in a minute, fewer objectives can be measured. On the other hand, matching and true–false questions make guessing possible. In terms of faculty time, matching and true–false questions take more time to write than short answer questions, but take less time to score.

The same three types of items can be used to test comprehension. But now a fourth type of item can be used: problem solving. By providing some data, faculty can ask students to demonstrate their use. While matching and true–false questions are not well–suited to test application objectives, short answer and problem solving as well as multiple choice items can be effective. Again, short answer and problem solving items may take more time to answer, so the number should be limited. But, students can respond to three multiple choice items per minute. Problem solving questions, like short answer questions, may take little time to write, but more time to grade. On the other hand, multiple choice questions, which are easy to score, are difficult to write.

Analysis and synthesis can be tested with essay questions as well as by short answer, problem solving, and multiple choice items. But, evaluation objectives can only be measured by the essay question. With essay questions, faculty can ask students to compare and contrast, establish relationships, analyze and synthesize information, draw implications, make conclusions, and take and defend positions. Of course, it would not be fair to test the students at the evaluation level with essay questions if the course objectives (and consequently the instruction) were set at lower levels. By matching the test to the objectives, we avoid first choosing a format and then limiting the test to only those objectives that can be measured with that format.

The fourth step in effective test writing is to draft test items, which leads directly to step five, pilot test with a colleague and revise if necessary. A colleague can help avoid embarrassing grammatical and spelling errors. When tests are developed by starting with step four, the course content covered may be unreliable and not valid. By unreliable, we mean that two students with the same overall content mastery may score differently. By invalid, we mean that teachers may not be evaluating what they want to evaluate. When faculty skip step five, they may inadvertently write items that are too easy or too difficult or that do not discriminate between high and low performers.

To check these characteristics, faculty should carry out a sixth, and last step: use the test results to analyze the test with difficulty and discrimination indices. These indices are calculated by comparing the top (27 percent) and the bottom (27 percent) students on each test item. The *difficulty index* is a measure of how the top and bottom groups together fared on the item. For example, let us suppose there are ten students in each group. If seven students in the top group and three in the bottom group answered the item correctly, the difficult index would be $(7 + 3) \div 20$ or .50. On the average, difficulty indices of fifty to seventy percent indicates that test items are not too hard or too easy.

The *discrimination index* is a comparison of the top and bottom groups on each item. In our example, this would be $7/10 - 3/10$ or .40. In general, the discrimination index should be at least .40. A negative discrimination index, which occurs when more students in the bottom group answer an item correctly than the students in the top group, may indicate that there is a problem with this question.

By taking time to follow these steps, medical school teachers can insure that their tests reflect their educational standards and measure student mastery. Yes, standardized tests such those constructed by the National Boards are important. But, those tests do not relieve faculty of their responsibility as the primary evaluators of student learning.

SUBJECT–BASED TEACHING

To help students achieve instructional **objectives**, teachers may break the subject down into topics and subtopics, with the intent of teaching the subject one part at a time. Such an approach is known as subject–based and is the traditional means of schooling from kindergarten though medical school, with a heavy emphasis on **lectures**. I am reminded of the grade school teacher announcing:

Good morning, class. Today I am going to tell

you how to read. Be sure to listen carefully, because I will be telling you many things that are very important about reading. *Ronald, close that book! How do you expect to learn how to read unless you pay attention to the teacher in reading class??*

Of course, subject–based teaching can be used with a **student–centered** rather than **teacher–centered learning** approach. In this design, the instructor leads a group discussion of topics. In either case, the main advantage of subject–based teaching versus **problem–based teaching** is that it helps teachers feel confident that they have thoroughly covered the important concepts. Of course, as I was once reminded in a workshop I was conducting on teaching skills, "Shouldn't we be trying to *uncover* material?"

This is a good point. Some teachers try to present too much material, which may result in less learning. It is important to remember that transmission does not equal reception. Effective use of this approach requires choosing the amount of material that students can learn in the amount of time provided. This principle was highlighted in a study conducted by Russell and colleagues (1984), in which one of the authors delivered three versions of a lecture on fibrositis to junior medical students. In the "low density" lecture, he spent 25 minutes on new material and 25 minutes on reinforcement (elaboration of the main points, reemphasis of prior concepts, and periodic summarizing). In the "medium density" lecture, he spent 35 minutes on new material and 15 minutes on reinforcement. In the "high density" lecture, he allocated 45 minutes to new material and 5 minutes to reinforcement.

Students were tested before the lecture, immediately after the lecture, and fifteen days later. The test consisted of sixteen questions that covered the content common to all three groups. There were no pre–lecture differences in test results. The "low density" group scored significantly higher than the "medium" and "high density" groups on the test given immediately after the lecture. Also, the "low density" group scored higher than the "high density" group fifteen days later. There was no statistical difference between the "low" and "medium" groups fifteen days later. In their analysis of which questions were answered incorrectly, the authors found that memory loss apparently was due to information presented later in the lecture displacing facts learned by students earlier in the same hour.

Despite test performance, a potential problem with the subject–based approach is that patients do not present as topics and subtopics. Ultimately, when students have to manage patients, they will find that each patient embodies many so–called "topics." A disadvantage of subject–based teaching is that students may have difficulty retrieving and applying the information they have learned. To overcome this difficulty, some medical schools, notably McMasters, Southern Illinois, New Mexico, and Harvard, rely upon problem–based teaching. These programs also emphasize a student–centered rather than teacher–centered approach to instruction.

TEACHER ABUSE

Although most medical faculty teach, the existing reward structure gives greater recognition to research, which leads to grants and promotion, and to service, which generates revenue. To some degree, the greater importance of research and service may be imposed by external demands to fund the medical school. To a larger degree, faculty themselves have created this reward structure through a system of peer approval. Noting that good teaching is neither fostered nor rewarded, Mark E. Saul, a winner of the National Science

Foundation Presidential Award for Excellence in Teaching, observed that teachers will teach the way they have been taught and that college teaching offers a poor role model for future teachers (1988).

Analyzing problems in medical education faced by students and teachers, Dr. Catherine P. McKegney, a faculty member at the University of Minnesota, suggested examining medical education as a system, just as patient problems can be understood by using a systematic approach to patients and their families. Using the **metaphor** of the family system, McKegney found the characteristics of neglectful and abusive families most applicable to the medical system (1989)!

According to McKegney's metaphor, who are the members of the medical education family? Department chairmen and senior faculty are the grandparents. Junior faculty, who are most responsible for teaching the next generation, are the parents. Senior residents function like late adolescents with concerns about impending independence, and interns are like school–age children concerned with proving their competence. Finally, medical students are the youngest siblings, uncertain and nervous about themselves.

Just as some adults who were victims of child abuse become abusers of their children, do some medical faculty perpetuate educational abuse they experienced as medical students and residents, including neglect of physical and emotional needs (see **student abuse**)? Certainly several studies reviewed by McKegney suggest that medical training produces high levels of **stress**. Since denial is a typical behavior of dysfunctional families, saying "it ain't so" reinforces McKegney's belief that medical education behaves as a dysfunctional family.

Having asked many medical students and residents about their educational experience, there is one abuse that I feel for sure has been passed down from generation to generation. This abuse begins early in the educational system: the lack of **feedback** that tells you what you are doing that is right and what can be improved. In addition, when we are given feedback, is it mostly negative? It is no wonder that today's medical teachers do not give adequate feedback to their students and residents, who are tomorrow's medical teachers. In this regard, I think that Dr. McKegney is on target:

> Negative judgment is common on all levels of medical education; direct feedback, which cites specifics and offers suggestions for improvement, is rare. Like adults who were scolded more than they were instructed as children, physicians have difficulty discerning the differences between describing behavior and labeling the person "good" or "bad." Because clear feedback is rare and correction is more common than affirmation, the medical trainee has difficulty feeling competent. Receiving punishing comments about mistakes teaches trainees to hide errors, by lying if necessary. Like emotionally abused children, residents become unwilling to risk the pain they have come to associate with close supervision. The absence of honest constructive feedback and the overabundance of placing blame in medical education perpetuate physicians' perfectionism and leave them at risk for impairment (p. 454).

TEACHER–CENTERED LEARNING

An important consideration in planning instruction is deciding who will be responsible for what is learned: the teacher or the student. Teacher–centered learning is the more traditional method because the instructor has the advantage of using his expertise to assure that all students will be exposed to the most important material. To use a photographic **metaphor**, the school is a camera and the students are rolls of film. By exposing students to the right amount of light (the level of content), controlling the depth of field (density of information) and focusing the camera (clarifying the details) the photographer (teacher) can take a picture (educate a student).

Of course, in this metaphor, the student plays as passive a role as a roll of film. The disadvantage is that students may not learn how to learn and do not acquire the skill of determining what is worth learning. This problem was discussed in *The School Book* by Postman and Weingartner (1980) who observed that, while teachers do most of the reading, writing, talking, and thinking, students take notes (see **note–taking**), "which is a hell of an activity for training stenographers, but not much good for anything else." One medical school teacher noticed the same phenomenon, commenting that the students' role was passive, "often consisting of listening and trying to decipher what I was trying to say during the lecture" (Glassman 1980, p. 31).

Whether combined with **subject–based teaching** (organizing the material around topics and subtopics) or **problem–based teaching** (organizing the presentation around patient cases), the teacher makes most of the decisions in teacher–centered learning. To educate medical students and residents for the next century, we must develop **student–centered learning**, *i.e.*, approaches that allow students to decide what is to be learned. After all, they are going to have to make these decisions eventually. Or, as one award–winning teacher once put it, "The true physician

never graduates from medical school; he simply transfers"
(Smith 1985).

TEACHER EVALUATION

Three aspects of faculty performance are evaluated for
the purposes of advancement and promotion: teaching,
research, and service. Service is considered a catch–all
category which rarely attracts attention as a bone of conten-
tion, except for clinical faculty who are required to generate
a portion of their salary with patient care revenue. On the
other hand, teaching and research are often seen as compet-
ing obligations. Implicit in the teaching–research dichotomy
is the widespread belief that teaching is relegated to a
second–class status because teaching is not rewarded in the
promotion process (see **faculty development strategies**).

The lack of interest in teaching medical students and
residents was explained by Dr. Richard M. Ratzan, who
asked, "Who would want to explain for the 50th time the
distribution of body water or diuretic–induced pre–renal
azotemia to an intern when one could be planning a research
project on the effect of antidiuretic hormone on microtu-
bules with a fellow over coffee and danish?" (1982, p. 1420)

One reason teaching is not given more weight is that
it is difficult to evaluate. This view is typified by one medical
educator: "If only you could give the promotions committee
more data about the candidate's teaching, we would be glad
to use it" (Rippey 1981, p.24). Admittedly, teacher evaluation has been problematic. As summed up by one reviewer...

> Systematic, comprehensive, and valid evalu-
> ation of teaching has been an educational
> problem for years. It continues to evade
> educators, although most administrators de-

sire it as a meaningful way to determine rewards and sanctions for faculty, and most serious teachers seek it as a way of improving their performance and more closely relating what they do to what students learn. Most evaluations of teaching have resulted in unfair and inconclusive distinctions among teachers without establishing reliable or valid relationships between what teachers do and what students learn (Meeth 1976, p. 3).

Unfortunately, many administrators and faculty equate teacher evaluation to **student ratings**. While students can tell us something important about teaching, *i.e.*, how they experienced the instruction, this is only one aspect of teaching. Other factors to be considered include colleague evaluation of teaching performance and teaching materials and student learning outcomes. Admittedly, evaluation of teaching is difficult. But, evaluation of research also would be difficult if not for refereed journals which do our research evaluation for us! What we need is more attention to *qualitative* objectivity (how good are the data collected?) and *quantitative* objectivity (how many sources of data are used?) (Whitman and Weiss 1982).

TEACHER TRAINING

Good teaching is an act of generosity, a whim of wanton muse, a craft that may grow with practice, and always risky business (Palmer 1990, p. 11).

Some teachers believe that good teachers are born, not made. This belief is not held only by poor teachers looking for excuses. Some very good teachers also think that little can be done to help improve teaching. In a survey of over 200 medical school **teaching award winners**, a medical student and I asked, "In your opinion, to what extent are teachers born (_____%) or made (_____%)?" We found that forty percent think that more than 50% of teaching expertise is made, and forty percent think that more than 50% is born. Twenty percent think it is 50/50 (Whitman and Ferrey).

My own belief is reflected in the title of my handbook on lecturing for medical teachers, *There Is No Gene for Good Teaching* (1982). My view notwithstanding, if medical teachers believe that little can be done to improve teaching, then teacher training will be seen as a waste of time. Certainly, the experience of many medical teachers with teacher training may reinforce this view. In many medical schools, the professional support for teacher training is located in an Office of Research in Medical Education. If, as the office name indicates, the primary objective is to study medical education rather than improve it, then teacher training may receive little attention. When it is addressed, it may be viewed only as an object of research.

Based on a survey of Offices of Research in Medical Education conducted in 1979 and repeated in 1983, Grovner, Smith and Schimpfhauser reported a decline in the percent of effort devoted to professional staff by teaching, instructional development, and educational support services, and a simultaneous shift from education to research. The authors concluded that educational specialists may be responding to the same forces that encourage medical faculty to shift attention from teaching to research.

Where educational services are provided, do medical faculty view them as helpful? Given the number of years medical teachers have spent in the educational system, they may be skeptical that "professional educators" can tell them anything about teaching. One such skeptic, Dr. Joseph D. Sapira, from the Department of Medicine at the St. Louis University School of Medicine, commented that key principles of medical education were "conspicuous by (their) absence from the writings and actions of most of our contemporary self–announced, self–certified, and self–serving medical 'educators' "(1986, p. 1141). This view is reinforced when Ph.D. educators cannot relate educational theory to clinical teaching, or when M.D. educators limit their prescription to personal, anecdotal experience. The challenge here is to provide teacher training activities that relate theory to practice and practice to theory.

Even in the best of circumstances, teaching teachers to teach is not easy. In fact, Carl Rogers commented that he could not teach another person how to teach! Basically, I think that learning to teach is like learning to write. There are two steps to learn to write: (1) Read. (2) Write. Similarly, I think there are two steps to learn to teach: (1) Learn. (2) Teach.

By *learn*, I mean paying attention to how you learn. Whenever you are in the role of learner, be aware of your own mental processes and what conditions facilitate your own learning. By *teach*, I mean that teaching is learned through practice. What you learn about teaching from learning and teaching will be increased if you become a **connoisseur** of teaching, *i.e.*, paying attention to what works and does not work.

Teacher training can improve teaching. There are specific, learnable skills to improve the **lecture** and **group discussions** (classroom teaching) as well as **morning report**, **teaching rounds,** and teaching at the **bedside** (clinical teaching). But, just as you cannot make a student learn (see **motivation**), I cannot make you become a better teacher. Teaching is like sex…if you don't like to do it, you won't be much good at it.

TEACHER'S ROLE

In its original meaning, a "professor" was not someone with esoteric knowledge and technique. Instead, the word referred to a person able to make a profession of faith...(Palmer 1990, p.16)

How teachers view themselves affects the way they teach. In response to the question, "What do you teach?", an Internist could say, "Internal Medicine" or "Medical students and residents." The former implies a relationship between a teacher and subject, the latter between a teacher and learners. Another way of looking at your role is to ask whether you see yourself as a medical library or as a medical librarian. The former suggests a fund of knowledge and the latter a guide to knowledge. To help you think about your role as a medical teacher, here are some statements about teaching and learning. Do any of these match your views about the **teaching–learning process**?

1. "Education should be gentle and stern, not cold and lax" (Joseph **Joubert**).

2. "Without discussion, intellectual experience is only an exercise in a private gymnasium" (Randolph Bourne).

3. "The true teacher defends his pupils against his own personal experience" (A. Bronson Alcott).

4. "The true physician never graduates from medical school, he simply transfers" (Lloyd Smith).

5. "Supposing is good, but finding out is better" (Mark Twain).

6. "Education is turning things over in the mind" (Robert Frost).

7. "A good teacher is one whose spirit enters the soul of the pupil" (John Milton).

8. "To spend too much time in studies is sloth" (Francis Bacon).

TEACHING

Carl Rogers once said that he could not teach anybody anything; he could only provide an environment in which **learning** could occur. Although most of us believe that teachers should play a more active role, this statement is a reminder that the purpose of teaching is to make learning possible. Of course, people can learn without teachers, and some medical students and residents say they learn despite the efforts of the medical school.

Studies of college teachers show that professors talk a lot. In fact, in typical classes, teachers are found talking 80% of the time. They also spend little time asking questions, typically less than 4% of the time. Medical teachers do a little better. They ask questions as much as 7% of the time (Ellner and Barnes). One medical school teacher noted that when he taught, he was the one who learned most: "I was the one whose thinking skills were enhanced and whose creativity was stimulated. I played the active learning role; the student's role was passive, often consisting of listening and trying to decipher what I was trying to say during the lecture" (Glassman, p. 31).

A problem for medical school teachers is that they and their students are products of an educational system in which teachers present information prepackaged and prewrapped (see **teacher abuse**). Students rarely learn how to analyze and synthesize material for themselves because they usually are dealing with the end product (Lindsey, Jr.).

This problem was highlighted for me when I saw a hematologist make what I thought was a brilliant effort to teach pathology.

He asked sophomore medical students to invent blood. He tried unsuccessfully to get the students to brainstorm all the characteristics of an ideal product that could circulate through the vascular system. For example, it should be a fluid that will clot if exposed to the external environment. The teacher's plan was to take the characteristics identified by the students and explain what can go wrong. I thought this was a **novel** way to teach pathology. The students were totally nonresponsive. They sat ready to take notes. They were waiting for him to teach. I hope that this teacher did not feel discouraged. It may take more than one effort to reach the students.

Good teaching practice includes encouraging student–faculty interaction, cooperation among students, and active learning. It means giving students prompt feedback on their performance and communicating high expectations (Chickering and Gamson). This does not preclude delivering information, but when they give information, creative teachers try to convey its "inner relevance" (Kestin). They seek to inspire, not just inform. One biologist aimed to persuade learners, "not just that the Darwinian worldview happens to be true, but that it is the only known theory that could, in principle, solve the mystery of our existence" (Dawkins)! Do you approach your subject with this vim and vigor?

To encourage you to practice good teaching, I would like to share the five principles of teaching recommended by John A. Rassias, the maverick professor of romance languages at Dartmouth College (Hechinger 1980a).

1. *Self–knowledge*: Look back at your own experience and learn from what did and did not work when you

were a student (see **connoisseurship**).

2.   *Direction*: Have goals and **objectives**, but be prepared for anything that may develop.

3.   *Spontaneity*: Do not transmit just what is in the text-book. Create the "illusion of the first time." After all, it is the first time…for the student (see **Raimi**).

4.   *Stage presence*: Be aware that not only the teacher, but also the student, can be a star (see **peer teaching**).

5   *The creative state*: Face the class intent on creating and sharing experiences. Students are more likely to remember something when their emotions as well as their intellect are engaged (see **remembering**).

TEACHING AWARD WINNERS

You can't win if you don't enter (Ed McMahon for Publisher's Clearinghouse).

A medical student and I surveyed 352 teaching award winners from 85 medical schools to discover their views of teaching (Whitman and Ferrey). Based on responses from 222 (63%), we found that the majority are senior faculty: 53% are full professors and 38% are associate professors. They have been teaching an average of 17 years and three out of four had won a teaching award more than once. Over half (56%) identified themselves as clinicians versus basic scientists (44%).

With regard to types of teaching, only 15% spent more than 50% of their time **lecturing**; however, only 3.7% reported no lecturing. Compared to lecturing, the respondents spent far less time leading **group discussions**; in fact 25% reported no group discussions. In general, clinical faculty spent most of their teaching time in **teaching rounds**, **morning report**, and teaching at the **bedside**.

According to these teaching award winners, the most important characteristic of effective lecturing concerned organization: effective lecturers present material in a clear and organized fashion, emphasizing major concepts and highlighting key points. They deliver lectures with enthusiasm and energy. They deem it important to present current issues in their field and to limit the amount of information. In leading group discussions, they emphasize group involvement and view the leader's role as a facilitator, asking questions, inviting comments, and allowing an exchange of ideas.

In the clinical setting, these teachers stressed the importance of discussing current developments and practical applications. They take the time to listen to student presentations and to ask the students to interpret, analyze, and evaluate patient data. Also, they remarked that clinical teachers should not humiliate students and engage in **pimping**.

Their largest motivation for teaching is the reward of seeing students learn. What they most like about teaching by far is seeing students learn, grow, "light up." What they dislike most is the lack of recognition for teaching and students who are not motivated. What they find most difficult is preparing for lectures and staying energetic when teaching the same subject over and over. Roughly three out of four respondents find **student ratings** helpful.

Medical school teaching award winners serve as role models for both students and faculty. Faculty who wish to become **connoisseurs** of teaching should find opportunities to observe the teaching award winners in their school and learn about teaching from their practices.

TEACHING–LEARNING PROCESS

Much I have learned from my teachers, more from my
colleagues, most from my students. (The Talmud)

The relationship between **teaching** and **learning** was
called into question by a cartoon in which a boy told his
friend that he had taught his dog how to whistle. With his
ear up to the dog's face, the friend said, "I don't hear him
whistling." The boy replied, "I said I taught him. I didn't say
he learned it."

My position is that if the learner didn't learn, then the
teacher didn't teach. In other words, teaching is analogous to
giving. By definition, if something is given, something is
received. If something is taught, something is learned.
Notwithstanding my view, some teachers are more comfortable with the view that teaching is analogous to *offering*.
When something is offered, it may or may not be received.
When something is taught, it may or not be learned.
Teachers who take the position that teaching is like offering
explain that if it was not the teacher's fault that learning did
not occur, then it would not be fair to say that the teacher
did not teach. I believe that, in the absence of learning, we
could say without assigning blame that the teacher did not
teach. By looking at teaching as giving, we focus on whose
performance really counts—the learner's rather than the
teacher's. The teacher might put on a good show or a poor
one, either of which may be long remembered. But to focus
on his performance confuses instructional means with
educational ends (Erickson, 1980).

I was reminded of this issue when I asked
anesthesiologists to evaluate my workshop on teaching skills.
The workshop had been conducted at the semi–annual
meeting of the Society for Education in Anesthesiology on
March 3, 1989. Participants were asked to re–evaluate the

workshop on May 1, 1989 (I provided stamped, self–addressed postcards—see **rating forms**). They were instructed to use as their criterion "the most exciting, personally rewarding, attention holding learning experience in your life." One person, who had rated the workshop a five on a seven point scale, did not return the follow–up postcard until August 19. He did not indicate a rating, but wrote:

"Now, five months later without specific review, I remember that I found the session stimulating, enjoyable, provoking, and clearly worth reviewing. But, in fact, I haven't reviewed it and can't recall any detail at this writing. My fault of course."

My point is that, regardless of fault, this person did not learn. Hence, I did not teach him! Of course, one could say there is always *something* being learned. In this anesthesiologist's case, we could say he learned that I was an entertaining instructor. While I may not mind making that impression, this was not the lesson I had planned. The fact is that every experience does teach something, whether it was the teacher's intention or not. Here I am reminded of another cartoon in which a boy tells his dad that a policeman gave a talk at school about safety and afterwards let the kids ride in his patrol car. The father asked what he had learned, and the boy replied that the siren button was under the dashboard.

Both teacher and learner play an important role in the **teaching–learning process**. As described by one professor of psychology, the best teachers are those who involve students so they learn as much as they can and think about the subject on their own, without the presence of the teacher (Lowman). While you cannot *make* students learn, you can *help* them learn. Since the skills of teaching are helping skills, effective teachers are, whether they realize it or not, specialists in human relations. A pioneer in the field of adult education, Leland Bradford, recognized that teachers bring more than knowledge to the teaching–learning process: they bring an awareness that it is basically a delicate human transaction, requiring skill and sensitivity in human relations.

The important relationship between teacher and learner was underscored by Carl Rogers who emphasized the teacher's role as a facilitator of learning. Many clinical teachers instinctively use the strategy of making the student responsible for his own learning because they realize that patient responsibility is an essential ingredient of clinical care. I would remind physician teachers that **clinical teaching is like clinical care** in that their role is to help another person. This view of teacher as helper was emphasized by one adult educator who noted that "program learnability" depends upon helping learners (1) become motivated to change, (2) handle new information and experience, (3) develop new knowledge, attitude, and skills, and (4) transfer their learning to new situations (McLagan 1978).

The teaching and learning process is a collaborative venture which depends upon an agreement between teachers and learners to work together toward common educational **objectives**. Certain attitudes seem essential to the success of this collaborative interaction. In a study of the influence of student feedback on **clinical teaching**, Tiberius *et al.* found that students respond much more enthusiastically to teachers who are genuinely interested in and committed to teaching them and teachers respond much more enthusiastically to students whom they perceive as eager to learn. "Interest, concern, commitment, enthusiasm, and eagerness are what make the process worthwhile for *all* the participants" (1989, p. 679).

Metaphors can clarify the teaching–learning interaction. Perhaps the most famous educational metaphor was invented by Socrates who said that the teacher was a midwife to students pregnant with ideas. Similarly, Wales and Stager, advocates of "**student–centered**" instruction, have stated:

> (Students) must learn what questions to ask, what questions not to ask, and when to ask. To learn in a meaningful way, they must teach themselves. The teacher can anticipate their problems, their concerns, but no teacher can learn for the student.... The teacher is not an intellectual surgeon implanting a pacemaker in the student's brain, but rather a midwife who assists in the delivery of a free mind.

The neurosurgeon metaphor was also used by Donald Norman, a cognitive psychologist, who warned against assuming that you can walk into a classroom, unscrew the tops of students' skulls, peer intently into the brain of each student, and say something like, "Hmmm, you seem to have that connection missing," and then proceed to rewire circuits.

Overall, there are few human functions more complex than the teaching–learning process, and even the most creative teachers may find humbling the attempt to help someone learn. One award–winning teacher acknowledged:

> How students learn and how teachers teach are complicated processes, difficult to understand and even harder to master. It is not surprising that professors of many years experience feel they have never quite got it right, and are amazed and gratified when the will to learn and the desire to teach come together in a few moments of excitement, pleasure, and joyful discovery (Schwartz).

TEACHING MODELS

For a physician or a medical student, a view of a patient's retina is like taking a tour at a world's fair. There, in miniature, in one place are representative samples of key body tissues. Blood vessel wall diseases, such as microaneurysm, are on display as are columns of blood choked with cholesterol emboli or optic nerves waterlogged from an expanding brain (Miller 1981, p. 671).

Dr. David Miller, a teacher of ophthalmology at Harvard Medical School, expressed concern that medical students are taught to explore this rich terrain by purchasing an expensive halogen ophthalmoscope, listening to one or two orientation lectures generally consisting of 50 to 100 **slides** of retinal diseases, and attending a session where one or two students have their eyes dilated while the rest of the class lines up for a look. Only for students who take an elective in ophthalmology does the ophthalmoscope convert from an expensive flashlight to a useful clinical tool!

The teaching model is a type of **simulation**. Dr. Miller constructed an eye teaching model to simulate the features found in the eye of a real patient. Glossy prints of retinal pictures representing systemic and ocular conditions such as retinal vein occlusion with papilledema and retinal artery occlusion were used to simulate the reflections. The retinal pictures were fitted into a two–ounce white jar, close to its center. Two pupillary apertures of 6 mm and 4 mm diameters were drilled in the screwtop of the jar, close to the center. A scratched piece of acetate, representing an immature cataract, was glued under the 4 mm pupil. The students first looked through the 6 mm "clear pupil" and then through the 4 mm "cataract." To further simulate reality, a piece of clear acetate was fitted into the screwtop jar cover, just under the pupillary apertures, to produce the annoying corneal reflection found in real patients.

Students hold the teaching model against a wall surface and aim the light of the ophthalmoscope into the pupillary apertures, moving to within an inch of the jar cover and turning the focus wheel until the retina comes into focus. As students become more proficient, they are asked to stop supporting the eye model against the wall and to simply hold it at eye level.

In addition to venous and arterial occlusions, other simulated conditions include hypertensive retinopathy, nonproliferative diabetic retinopathy, retinitis pigmentosa, retinal detachment, choridial melanoma, and proliferative diabetic retinopathy. Follow–up interviews with students indicated they were able to see these conditions in patients on the hospital wards. Thus, with some creative thinking, a **novel** and **useful** teaching model enhanced the learning process.

TEACHING ROUNDS

When a team is finished with **morning report**, the attending physician, residents, and students typically leave the conference room and pass by each patient's room. I say "pass by" because they often do not enter the patient's room. In any case, whether or not there is true **bedside teaching**, there almost always is a discussion in the hallway outside the patient's room. Having followed these teams in many hospitals, I have learned how to find the soft spot on the wall and settle in for five or ten minutes of "teaching," while nursing aides wheel by with breakfast trays, nurses push the medication cart down the corridor, technicians arrive to collect specimens or take the patients to radiology, patients take their morning stroll, and family members arrive to visit their loved ones. Meanwhile, ward team members drop in and out, answering pages and talking with nurses. In the midst of this chaos, the ward team may engage in serious discussion of confidential matters!

To make teaching rounds more effective, Weinholtz (1977) suggests that attending physicians limit the time spent in the hallway. Spend as much time as possible at the bedside, demonstrating ways of discovering physical findings and observing team members' efforts to discover these, themselves.

According to Stritter (1983), there are a number of ways to improve teaching skills on rounds, including being observed by an educational consultant and participating in collaborative educational research. In 1981, Dr. Thomas L. Schwenk used me as his consultant to improve his teaching rounds. Dr. Schwenk and I adapted the AIMS (Advanced Instruction to Medical Settings) model developed by the University of Kentucky College of Medicine, in which the assessment and improvement of instruction parallels the physician–patient encounter. Applying this analogy, the educational consultant takes a "history" of the instructor's teaching experience and conducts a "physical examination" of current teaching practices. The consultant also collects "laboratory" data regarding the instructor's performance, such as resident ratings. Based on "historical, physical, and laboratory" findings, the consultant "diagnoses" the instructor's teaching problems and "treats" the instructor with recommended changes in teaching rounds.

As a result of their experience, Whitman and Schwenk (1982) found that evaluation can improve teaching rounds if...

1.   resident ratings are combined with educational consultation;

2.   the teacher compares resident ratings to self–ratings;

3. evaluations are collected early enough to give the teacher time to improve; and

4. the teacher's efforts to improve are rewarded.

TECHNIQUES

Whereas **methods** of teaching refer to the relationship between the teacher and the learner, techniques of teaching refer to procedures and processes used by the teacher. For example, the lecture is a teaching *method* in which the teacher is active and the learner is passive. **Questioning** is a teaching *technique* in which the teacher elicits answers from students. Not all techniques can be used appropriately with all methods, but some are useful with many methods. For example, according to Kidd (1973), both the **lecture** and the **group discussion** (methods) could use **brainstorming** (technique).

Techniques comprise an armamentarium which the teacher uses to make the chosen teaching method effective. For example, you may choose to lecture because there are low level **knowledge** objectives (facts and comprehension) you want the students to achieve. In the lecture method, the teacher is actively presenting information and the student is in the passive role of listening. If no techniques are used to encourage mental involvement by students, little learning may occur. So, techniques can be used to encourage a more active role. Conversely, you may choose the group discussion method because there are higher level knowledge objectives you want the students to achieve (application, analysis, synthesis, or evaluation) or you want to effect **attitudinal change.** In the group discussion method, both the teacher and the learners share an active role. If no techniques are used to encourage student participation, little learning may occur. So, techniques can be used to encourage students to talk and listen to each other.

Three techniques can be used in both lectures and group discussions: questioning, brainstorming, and **demonstrations.** Two additional techniques are appropriate to group discussions, but may not be feasible in lectures: **role playing** and **simulations.** Using these techniques can provide an opportunity for teachers to be creative.

For example, I worked with a faculty member who was planning a group discussion with faculty colleagues on the topic of "drug issues in the community." By brainstorming during our planning session, we developed a technique in which each participant received a letter in the mail in advance of the group discussion concerning a group of high school students found smoking marijuana on school grounds, after school hours. This letter came from the school principal. Each faculty member, except one, was addressed in the letter as a parent of one of these students. One faculty member was instructed that he would play the role of the principal who had sent the letters. The principal's letter invited the parents to a meeting to discuss what should be done. Each faculty member readily accepted the role of "parent" or "principal" and, as you can imagine, a lively discussion was conducted which elicited many drug issues in the community. One parent even brought his "lawyer."

When you use a teaching technique, or when you are the recipient of a teaching technique, pay attention to whether it works well and how it could be improved in another setting. This process of attending to the effectiveness of teaching is known as **connoisseurship**.

USEFUL

In the hundreds of medical lectures I have attended, I suspect that almost all the information was correct and that most of it was up–to–date. When a medical lecture is not useful, the problem usually lies with the information being irrelevant to the learners. The question for a creative teacher is, "What do my learners need to know?" The tendency is to cover too much material. In one of my workshops on lecture skills, a participant commented, "Isn't our real goal to *uncover* the material?" I think that was a perceptive comment; a corollary of creative teaching is that teachers who are useful uncover rather than cover material.

Defining teaching as "a process of information trans-mission" does not adequately describe what occurs in class-room or clinical settings. In a study of evaluative feedback in clinical teaching, Tiberius *et al.* (1989) found that the teach-ers rated highest by medical students were those judged as having the greater number of personal attributes such as warmth, sensitivity, and accessibility. Moreover, faculty identified the importance of **enthusiasm** and commitment as key factors in their improvement of teaching. Yet, the chief concern of some medical teachers is that they do not give enough information.

Why do medical teachers try to cover too much information? One reason is due to the "information anxiety" that pervades medicine today. Information anxiety is pro-duced by the ever–widening gap between what we under-stand and what we think we should understand (Wurman 1989). When medical teachers become anxious over the gap between what students know and what they should know, they try to lessen the gap by transmitting more information. The problem with this approach is that students may not receive the information. In the face of **information overload**, some students stop learning. In one study of medical student retention of information, the investigators found that the students remembered more essential informa-tion in a low–density lecture on fibrositis that amplified the basics than in a high–density lecture that tried to cover the field (Russell, Hendricson, and Herbert 1984).

Of course, high versus low density is a matter of perception. The difference in perception was highlighted by a story in the *Los Angeles Times*. According to Franklin R. Garfield, he has difficulty playing the "word of the day" game with his teenage daughter. It's a simple game. Every day he gives her a new word and expects her to look it up in the dictionary, learn it, and use it. On most days, their conversation goes something like this:

—"Sweetheart, it's only one word a day."

—"But, Dad, I have lots of other things to do, you know. I don't have time for this too."

Garfield persists and she resists. She even has an educational principle to support her position: "the more she learns, the more she forgets." If education is what's left over after she's forgotten what she learned, maybe she is right. This learning theory was described by one teacher of Anesthesiology as the "queuing theory" (see **Cook's Learning Theories**):

> These lecturers suppose that the student has a limited memory for a subject, consisting of a finite number of slots that contain simple data items. Slots are arranged in a queue and data may be put into and later retrieved from the queue according to a set of rules.

> Most lecturers who use queueing theory believe in a last–in first–out (LIFO) queue rule (the most recently learned data item is the first to be recalled). Overflow of the queue, according to the theory, causes loss of the

oldest data. These lecturers compete for lecture hours immediately preceding examinations.

In contrast, a small group of lecturers believe in the first–in first–out (FIFO) method of queueing. They believe that overflow of the queue causes new items to be lost and that permanence in memory is a function of early presentation. They schedule lectures early in the term (Cook 1989).

The fact is that, regardless of the order in which facts are presented, students will remember what they understand, they will understand what they pay attention to, and they will pay attention to what they want. Teachers who are useful give students reasons for listening. They make what students listen to understandable and, hence, memorable (see **remembering**). As noted by Dr. John Stone, who teaches cardiology at Emory University Medical School, memory is part of a long biochemical *and* emotional equilibrium. It is on one side of a balanced equation that has "forgetting" on the other side. Part of a student's struggle, like Garfield's daughter, is to remember what he needs to remember and to forget what is worth forgetting. Stone calls this phenomenon a "felicitous equilibrium" (1989).

WAIT TIMES

By remaining silent when a learner pauses, a teacher can communicate that he understands what has been said. By remaining silent after asking a question, the teacher provides the student with time to think. Unfortunately, many teachers find it difficult to remain silent. When they ask a question, they are too quick to repeat it or answer it themselves. Videotapes of university teachers revealed an average wait time of less than two seconds after professors asked questions (Rowe 1974). If you remain silent for three to five seconds after asking a question, you provide students time to think. By remaining silent for a few seconds *after* a student has responded, you provide him an opportunity to add to his answer. Also, if this encounter takes place in a small group setting, you give other students a chance to assess the answer.

Some skydiving instructors tell their students to take a breath and repeat the words, "Not now, but now," when they think it is time to pull the parachute cord. This is good advice for teachers when they think it is time to talk. Take a breath and repeat those words before you commence. This technique extends the wait time just a little, hence providing students time to think. Some teachers like to use the **coffee cup** technique to extend their wait times. Whatever strategy you use, please give students enough time to respond to your questions and assess the answers of others.

References

Abrahamson, Stephen. "Myths and Shibboleths in Medical Education." *Teaching and Learning in Medicine* 1(1): 4–9, 1989.

Abrami, Phillip C., Leventhal, Les, and Perry, Raymond. "Educational Seduction." *Review of Educational Research* 52: 446–463, 1982.

Aleamoni, Lawrence M. "Typical Faculty Concerns about Student Evaluation of Teaching." *New Directions for Teaching and Learning* 31: 25–31, 1987.

Altman, Lawrence K. "The Doctor's World: Med Schools under Attack." *The New York Times*: 21, June 22, 1982.

Anderson, J. and Graham, A. "A Problem in Medical Education: Is There an Information Overload?" *Medical Education* 14: 4–7, 1980.

Anderson, Scarvia B. "Tests that Stand the Test of Time." *The New York Times Education Supplement*: 61, 1987.

Association of American Medical Colleges, Clinical Evaluation Project. "The Evaluation of Clerks: Perceptions of Clinical Faculty." 1983.

Association of American Medical Colleges. "Physicians for the Twenty–First Century." *The Journal of Medical Education* 59(11): 1984.

Baldwin, DeWitt C., Jr. *et al.* "The Experience of Mistreatment and Abuse among Medical Students." presented at the Research in Medical Education Proceedings, Association of American Medical Colleges, Chicago, November 11, 1988.

Bateman, Kim A. "Rural Preceptorship: A Personal Perspecive." *Utah Medical Association Bulletin* 35(7): 10–11, 1987.

Best, Judith. "Teaching Political Theory: Meaning through Metaphor." *Improving College and University Teaching* 32: 165–168, 1984.

Betcher, R. William. *A Student to Student Guide to Medical School: Study Strategies, Mnemonics, Personal Growth.* New York: Little Brown and Company, 1985.

Bibace, Roger *et al.* "Teaching Styles in the Faculty–Resident Relationship." *The Journal of Family Practice* 13(6): 895–900, 1981.

Billings, J. Andrew *et al.* "A Seminar in 'Plain Doctoring.' " *The Journal of Medical Education* 60(11): 855–859, 1985.

Bishop, F. Marian. "Preceptorships in the 21st Century." *Utah Medical Association Bulletin* 35(6): 12, 14, 1987.

Bishop, J. Michael. "Infuriating Tensions: Science and the Medical Student." *Journal of Medical Education* 59(2): 91–102, 1984.

Blanchard, Kenneth and Johnson, Spencer. *The One Minute Manager.* New York: William Morrow and Company, 1982.

Bland, Carole J. *Faculty Development though Workshops.* Springfield, IL: Charles C. Thomas Publisher, 1980.

Bloom, Benjamin *et al. Taxonomy of Educational Objectives: Handbook I. Cognitive Domain.* New York: David McKay, 1956.

Bojar, S. "Psychiatric Problems of Medical Students." In *Emotional Problems of the Student*, edited by G.B. Blaine, Jr. and C.C.McArthur. New York: Appleton–Century–Crofts, 1971.

Bolles, Edmund Blair. *Remembering and Forgetting: Inquiries into the Nature of Memory.* New York: Walker and Company, 1988.

Bradford, Leland. "The Teaching–Learning Transaction." *Adult Education* 8(3): 135–145, 1958.

Brancati, Frederick L. "The Art of Pimping." *The Journal of the American Medical Association* 262(1): 89–90, 1989.

Bronowski, Jacob. *The Visionary Eye: Essays in the Arts, Literature, and Science*. Cambridge: The MIT Press, 1978.

Bruffee, Kenneth. "Collaborative Learning and 'The Conversation of Mankind.' " *College English* 46(6):635–652, 1984.

Bruner, Jerome. *The Process of Education*. Cambridge: Harvard University Press, 1966.

Bunnell, Kevin, editor. *Continuing Medical Educator's Handbook*. Denver: Colorado Medical Society, 1980.

Bunnell, Kevin. "The Difference between Teacher–Centered Teaching and Learner–Centered Teaching." presented at the Alliance for Continuing Medical Education, Miami, January 30, 1987.

Bursztajn, Harold *et al*. *Medical Choices, Medical Chances: How Patients, Families, and Physicians Cope with Uncertainty*. New York: Delacore Press, 1981.

Change Magazine. *Guide to Effective Teachers*. New York: Change Magazine Press, 1978.

Chickering, Arthur and Gamson, Zelda. "Seven Principles for Good Practice in Undergraduate Education." *The Wingspread Journal* 9(2): 1987.

Christian, Henry A. "Osler: Recollections of an Undergraduate Medical Student at Johns Hopkins." *Archives of Internal Medicine* 84: 77–83, 1949.

Clegg, Victoria L. and Owens, Richard E. *Tips for Writing Tests*. Manhattan, KS: Office of Educational Improvement, Kansas State University, 1983.

Collins, George F., Cassie, Josephine M., and Daggett, Christopher J. "The Role of the Attending Physician in Clinical Training." *Journal of Medical Education* 53(5): 429–431, 1978.

Cook, Richard I. "Learning Theories Implicit in Medical Lectures." *Journal of the American Medical Association* 261(15): 2244–2245, 1989.

Costin, F., Greenough, W., and Menges, R. "Student Ratings of College Teaching: Reliability, Validity, and Usefulness." *Review of Educational Research* 41: 511–535, 1971.

Cousteau, Voltaire. "How to Swim with Sharks." *Perspectives in Biology and Medicine* Summer: 525–528, 1973.

Crain, Ellen and Crain, William. "Clinical Impression." letter to the editor, *The Journal of Medical Education* 62(6): 539, 1987.

Cross, K. Patricia. "Teaching for Learning." *AAHE Bulletin* 39(8): 3–7, 1987.

Davis, Robert H., Fry, John P., and Alexander, Lawrence T. *The Discussion Method.* East Lansing: Michigan State University, 1977.

Dawkins, Richard. *The Blind Watchmaker.* New York: W. W. Norton and Company, 1987.

DeMott, Benjamin. "Knowing and Not Knowing." *Change* 21(5): 62, 1989.

Department of Family and Community Medicine. *Educational Objectives for Family Practice Residency.* Salt Lake City: University of Utah School of Medicine, 1975.

Detmer, Don, Fryback, Dennis, and Gassner, Kevin. "Heuristics and Biases in Medical Decision–Making." *Journal of Medical Education* 53: 682–683, 1978.

Divesta, F.J. and Gray, G.S. "Listening and Note–Taking," *Journal of Educational Psychology* 63: 8–14, 1972.

Dodge, W.T. "Communication and Interpersonal Skills." In *Fundamentals of Family Medicine*, edited by R.B. Taylor. New York: Springer–Verlag, 1983.

Dunn, Earl V., Norton, P.G., and Dunn, Ruth C. "Using Simulated Patients to Teach Family Practice Residents to Manage Patients by Telephone." *The Journal of Medical Education* 62(6): 524–526, 1987.

Eble, Kenneth. *The Craft of Teaching*, second edition. San Francisco: Jossey Bass Publishers, 1988.

Edwards, Janine and Marier, Robert, editors. *Resident Teaching: Rules, Techniques, and Programs.* New York: Springer Publishing Company, 1988.

Eichna, Ludwig W. "A Medical School Curriculum for the 1980s." *The New England Journal of Medicine* 308(1): 18–21, 1981.

Eichna, Ludwig W. "Medical School Education, 1975–1979." *The New England Journal of Medicine* 303(13): 727–734. 1980.

Eisner, Elliot. *The Educational Imagination.* New York: The Macmillian Publishing Company, 1979.

Ellner, Carolyn L. and Barnes, Carol P. *Studies of College Teaching.* Lexington, MA: Lexington Books, 1983.

Elstein, Arthur, Shulman, Lee S., and Sprafka, Sara. *Medical Problem Solving.* Cambridge: Harvard University Press, 1978.

Engel, George. "What if music students were taught to play their instruments as medical students are taught to interview?" *The Pharos* Fall: 12–13, 1982.

Erickson, Stanford. "The Motivation to Remember." *Memo to the Faculty.* Ann Arbor: Center for Research on Learning and Teaching, the University of Michigan, No. 67, December, 1980.

Evans, Mary. "The Abuse of Slides." *British Medical Journal*: 905–908, April 8, 1978.

Featherstone, H.J., Beitman, B.D., and Irby, D.M. "Distorted Learning from Unusual Anecdotes." *Medical Education* 18: 155–158, 1984.

Ficklin, Fred L. *et al.* "Faculty and House Staff Members as Role Models." *The Journal of Medical Education* 63(5): 392–396, 1988.

Foley, Richard P. and Smilansky, Jonathan. *Teaching Techniques: A Handbook for the Health Professions*. New York: McGraw Hill Book Company, 1980.

Foley, Richard P., Smilansky, Jonathan, and Yonke, A. "Teacher–Learner Interaction in a Medical Clerkship." *Journal of Medical Education* 54: 622, 1978.

Foster, Patricia. "Verbal Participation and Outcomes in Medical Education: A Study of Third–Year Clinical Discussion Groups." In *Studies of College Teaching*, edited by C.L. Ellner and C.P. Barnes. Lexington, MA: Lexington Books, 1983.

Francis, Robert. *Travelling in Amherst: A Poet's Journal*, 1930–1950. Amherst: The University of Massachusetts Press, 1985.

Friedlander, Myrna.L. and Phillips, Susan.D. "Preventing Anchoring Errors in Clinical Judgment. *Journal of Consulting and Clinical Psychology* 52: 366, 1984.

Frost, G.E. *Speech Communication for the Classroom Teacher*, edited by P.J. Cooper.

Frost, H.G. "Observations on a Great Occasion." *Adult Education* 37(5): 283, 1965.

Fuhrmann, Barbara Schneider and Grasha, Anthony F. *A Practical Handbook for College Teachers*. Boston: Little, Brown and Company, 1983.

Gabgan, Patricia. "Treating Computer Anxiety with Training." *Training and Development Journal*, July 1983.

Gaensbauer, Theodore J. and Mizner, George L. "Developmental Stresses in Medical Education." *Psychiatry* 43: 60–70, 1980.

Gary, Nancy E. "Barriers to Medical Student Education in Ambulatory Settings." *Journal of Medical Education* 62(6): 527–529, 1987.

Gil, Doran, Rubeck, Robert F., and Dinham, Sarah. "Parallels in the Medical and Educational Roles of the Physician–Teacher." *The Arizona Medical Educator* 13: June, 1981.

Glassman, Edward. "The Teacher as Leader." *New Directions for Teaching and Learning* 1: 31–40, 1980.

Gordon, Michael S. "Cardiology Patient Simulator." *American Journal of Cardiology* 34: 350–355, 1974.

Gordon, T. *Parent Effectiveness Training*. New York: Peter H. Wyden, 1970.

Gordon, T. *Teacher Efffectiveness Training*. New York: Peter H. Wyden, 1975.

Gregg, Alan. *For Future Doctors*. Chicago: University of Chicago Press, 1957.

Gronlund, Norman E. *Stating Objectives for Classroom Instruction*. New York: Macmillan Publishing Company, 1978.

Grovner, P.L., Smith, D.U., and Schimpfhauser, F. "Activities and Trends in Offices of Research in Medical Education." *Professional Educator Research Notes* 6: 3–6, 1985.

Guba, Egon G. and Lincoln, Yvonna S. *Effective Evaluation*. San Francisco: Jossey–Bass Publishers, 1981.

Harrington, Maura J. "Taking Surgery to a New Dimension." *Computerworld*: 16, May 21, 1990.

Harvard Medical School Office of Educational Development. "The New Pathway to General Medical Education at Harvard University." *Teaching and Learning in Medicine* 1 (1): 42–26, 1989.

Harvey, Richard F. *et al.* "Dreaming during Scientific Papers: Effects of Added Extrinsic Material." *British Medical Journal* 287: 1916–1919, 1983.

Hechinger, Fred M. "About Education: A Maverick Teacher Enlivens Students with Flair and Style." *The New York Times*: October 14, 1980a.

Hechinger, Fred M. "Extraordinary Teachers are Remembered." *The New York Times*: October 28, 1980b.

Higbee, Kenneth L. *Your Memory and How it Works*. Englewood Cliffs, NJ: Prentice–Hall, 1977.

Highet, George. *The Art of Teaching*. New York: Knopf, 1950.

Hirsch, S. Roger. "To the Editor." *The New England Journal of Medicine* 304(12): 738, 1981.

Hockey, Robert. "Stress and Cognitive Components of Skilled Performance." In *Human Stress and Cognition*, edited by V. Hamilton and D. Warbutin. New York: John Wiley and Sons, 1979.

Hollinger, Thomas G. "Problem–Based Learning in the Traditional Curriculum." presented at the Rsearch in Medical Education Proceedings, Association of American Medical Colleges, Washington, D.C., October 27, 1989.

Ingalsbe, N. and Spears, M.C. "Development of an Instrument to Evaluate Critical Incident Performance." *Journal of the American Dietetic Association* 74: 134–140, 1979.

Irby, David M. "Clinical Teacher Effectiveness in Medicine." *Journal of Medical Education* 53(10): 808–815, 1978.

Irby, David M. "Clinical Teaching and the Clinical Teacher." *The Journal of Medical Education* 61(9) Part 2: 35–45, 1986.

Irby, David M. and Dohner, Charles W. "Student Clinical Performance." in *Teaching in the Health Professions* by C.W. Ford and M. M. Morgan. St. Louis: C.V. Mosby, 1976.

Irby, David M. and Rakestraw, Phillip. "Evaluating Clinical Teaching in Medicine." *The Journal of Medical Education* 56(3): 181–186, 1981.

Irby, David M. *et al.* "The Use of Student Ratings in Multiinstructor Courses." *The Journal of Medical Education* 52(8): 668–673, 1977.

Irvine, William. *Apes, Angels, and Victorians.* New York: McGraw–Hill, 1955.

Israel, Lucien. *Decision–Making: The Modern Doctor's Dilemma.* New York: Random House, 1982.

Joubert, Joseph. *The Notebooks of Joseph Joubert,* edited and translated by Paul Auster. San Francisco: North Point Press, 1983.

Kahn, Henry S. "To the Editor." *The New England Journal of Medicine* 304(12): 738, 1981.

Kappel–Smith, Diana. *Night Life: Nature from Dusk to Dawn.* Boston: Little, Brown and Company, 1990.

Kassirer, Jerome P. "Teaching Clinical Medicine by Iterative Hypothesis Testing: Let's Preach What We Practice." *The New England Journal of Medicine* 309(15): 921–923, 1983.

Kaufman, Arthur *et al.* "The New Mexico Experiment: Educational Innovation and Institutional Change." *Academic Medicine* 64(6): 285–294, 1989.

Keller, John. "Strategies for Stimulating the Motivation to Learn." *Performance and Instruction* 26: 1–8, 1987.

Kern, Leslie. and Doherty, Michael.E. "Pseudodiagnosticity in an Idealized Medical Problem–Solving Environment." *Journal of Medical Education* 57(2): 100–104, 1982.

Kestin, John. "Creativity in Teaching and Learning." *American Scientist* 58: 250–257, 1970.

Kidd, J.R. *How Adults Learn.* New York: Association Press, 1973.

King, Thomas C. "Teaching the House Officer to Teach." *American College of Surgeons Bulletin*: 8–10, May, 1983.

Kirsling, Robert A. and Kochar, Mahendor S. "Mentors in Graduate Education at the Medical College of Wisconsin." *Academic Medicine* 65(4): 272–272, 1990.

Klass, Perri. "Facing up to 007's." *Discover*: 20–22, August, 1985.

Klass, Perri. *A Not Entirely Benign Procedure: Four Years as Medical Student.* New York: New American Library, 1987.

Knopke, Harry J. and Diekelman, Nancy L. *Approaches to Teaching in the Health Sciences.* Menlo Park: Addison–Wesley, 1978

Knowles, Malcolm. *The Modern Practice of Education.* New York: Association Press, 1970.

Knox, Alan. "Helping Teachers Help Adults Learn." *New Directions for Continuing Education* 6: 73–100, 1980.

Knudson, Mark P. "Analysis of Resident and Attending Physician Interactions in Family Medicine." *The Journal of Family Practice* 28(6): 705–709, 1989.

Konner, Melvin. *Becoming a Doctor.* New York: Penguin Books, 1987.

Kramer, Steven G. and Schwartz, Ariah. "In Support of Clearer Public Speaking." *American Journal of Ophthalmology*: 657–658, November, 1986.

Krathwohl, David R., Bloom, Benjamin S., and Masia, Bertram B. *Taxonomy of Educational Objectives, Handbook II: Affective Domain.* New York: David McKay Company, 1964.

Kravitz, Lee. "Future–Bound: Glimpses of Life in the 21st Century." *Scholastic Update*, December 1, 1986.

Kroenke, Kurt. "The Lecture: Where It Wavers." *The American Journal of Medicine* 77(3): 393–396, 1984.

Kuehl, LeRoy. "The Lecture Paradox." *The Pharos* 49(2): 32, 1986.

Kugel, Peter. "A Little Coffee to the Rescue." *The New York Times Education Life*: 78, January 8, 1989.

Kummer, Corby. "What Cooking Classes Teach." *The Atlantic Monthly*: 96–99, June, 1985.

Lamkin, B. Mygdal, W.K., and Hitchcock, M. "Perceptions of the Ideal Clinical Teacher: Views of Family Medicine Educators." *Family Practice Development Center of Texas* 4(1): 1–4, 1983.

Leary, Mark R. *et al.* "Boredom in Interpersonal Encounters: Antecedents and Social Implications." *Journal of Personality and Social Psychology* 51: 968–975, 1986.

Lenkai, Elaine J. and Bissonette, Raymond P. "A Useful and Cost–Effective Way to Provide Feedback from Students to Community–Physician Preceptors." *Academic Medicine* 64(1): 51, 1989.

Levinson, Daniel. *The Seasons of a Man's Life.* New York: Alfred A. Knopf, 1978.

Lindsey, Crawford W., Jr. *Teaching Students to Teach Themselves.* New York: Nichols Publishing, 1988.

Linfors, Eugene W. and Neelson, Francis A. "The Case for Bedside Rounds." *The New England Journal of Medicine* 303(21): 1230–1233, 1980.

Linfors, Eugene W. and Neelson, Francis A. "To the Editor." *The New England Journal of Medicine* 304(12): 738, 1981.

Lowman, Joseph. *Mastering the Techniques of Teaching.* San Francisco: Jossey–Bass Publishers, 1984.

Mager, Robert and Pipe, Peter. *Analyzing Performance Problems.* Belmont, CA: Fearon Publishers, 1970.

Mager, Robert. *Preparing Instructional Objectives.* Belmont, CA: Fearon Publishers, 1962.

Magnan, Robert. *147 Tips for Teaching Professors.* Madison: Magna Publications, Inc. 1989.

Mangione, C. M. "How Medical School Did and Did Not Prepare Me for Graduate Medical Education." *Journal of Medical Education* 61(9), Part 2: 3–10, 1986.

Margon, Marilyn. "Strengthening the Teaching Role in Residency Training." *Journal of the Medical Women Association* 34(2): 89–91, 1979.

McBeath, Ron J. and Lane, Janice, M. *Conducting Discussions.* San Jose: San Jose State University, 1977.

McGregor, Douglas. *Leadership and Motivation.* Cambridge: MIT Press, 1966.

McGuire, Christine H. "Medical Problem–Solving: A Critique of the Literature." *The Journal of Medical Education* 60(8): 587–594, 1985

McGuire, Christine H. and Wezeman, Frederick H. "Simulation in Instruction and Evaluation in Medicine." *World Health Organization Public Health Reports*, No. 60–703: 18–34, 1975.

McKegney, Catherine P. "Medical Education: A Neglectful and Abusive Family System." *Family Medicine* 21(6): 452–457, 1989.

McLagan, Patricia. *Helping Others Learn*. Reading, MA: Addison–Wesley Publishing Company, 1978.

McLeish, J. "The Lecture Method." In *The Psychology of Teaching Methods*, edited by N.L. Gage. Chicago: The University of Chicago Press, 1976.

Meeth, Richard. "The Stateless Art of Teaching Evaluation." *Change Report on Teaching* 2: 3–5, 1976.

Meichenbaum, Donald "The Clinical Potentials of Modifying What Clients Say to Themselves." In *Self–Control: Power to the Person*, edited by M. Mahoney and C. Thoreson. Monterey, CA: Brooks/Cole Publishing Company, 1974.

Miller, Charles F. "New Housestaff: Officers and Physicians." *Military Medicine* 155(April): 190, 1990.

Miller, David. "A Teaching Eye Model for Ophthalmoscopy." *The Journal of Medical Education* 56(8): 671–672, 1981.

Miller, George. *Education for the Future*. Chicago: National Society for the Study of Education, 1962.

Minsky, Marvin. *The Society of Mind*. New York: Simon and Schuster, 1985.

Mouw, David R. "Using the Personal (Very Personal) Anecdote." *New Directions for Teaching and Learning* 7: 27–30, 1981.

Naftulin, Donald H., Ware, John E., and Donnelly, Frank, A. "The Dr. Fox Lecture: A Paradigm of Educational Seduction." *The Journal of Medical Education* 48(7): 630–635, 1973.

Nash, Jim. "Bridging the Real and the Unreal." *Computer World*, March 12, 1990.

Ness, David E. "Short Stories about Doctor and Patients." *Academic Medicine* 64(7): 390, 1989.

Neufield, Victor R. *et al.* "Clinical Problem–Solving by Students: A Cross Sectional and Longitudinal Analysis." *Medical Education* 15: 515, 1981.

Norman, Donald. "What Goes on in the Mind of the Learner." *New Directions in Teaching and Learning* 2: 39, 1980.

Osborn, Alex F. *Applied Imagination.* New York: Scribner, 1963.

Osler, William. "On the Need of a Radical Reform in Our Methods of Teaching Senior Students." *The Medical News* 82: 49–52, 1903.

Overall, Jesse U. and Marsh, Herbert W. "Students' Evaluations of Teaching: An Update." *AAHE Bulletin* 35: 12, 1982.

Palmer, Parker J. "Good Teaching: A Matter of Living the Mystery." *Change* 22(1): 10–16, 1990.

Papper, S. "The Creative Clinician." *Archives of Internal Medicine* 144: 2049–2050, 1984.

Perkoff, Gary T. "Teaching Clinical Medicine in the Ambulatory Setting." *The New England Journal of Medicine* 314: 27–31, 1986.

Personnel Journal. "Conscious Competency — The Mark of a Competent Instructor." 538(7): 1974.

Petersdorf, Robert G. "From the President." *Academic Medicine* 65(1): 28, 1990.

Petrusa, Emil. "The Effect of Number of Cases on Performance on a Standardized Multiple–Station Clinical Examination." *The Journal of Medical Education* 62(10): 559–860, 1987.

Popham, W. James. "Instructional Objectives: 1960–1970." presented at the National Society for Programmed Instruction, Anaheim, May 1, 1970.

Postman, Neil and Weingartner, Charles. *The School Book*. New York: Delacorte Press, 1973.

Prial, Frank. "Accounting for Tastes." *The New York Times Magazine*: September 9, 1984.

Prichard, Robert W., Gardner, William A., Jr., and Anderson, H. Clarke. "Faculty Development in the Pathology Department: A 1988 Symposium of the Association of Pathology Chairmen." *Human Pathology* 20(9): 827–831, 1989.

Raimi, Ralph. "Twice–Told Tale—The Joy of Teaching." *The New York Times Spring Survey of Education*: 59, April 26, 1981.

Ramsey, Ruthanne and Whitman, Neal. *A Problem–Based, Student–Centered Approach to Teaching Geriatrics in the Classroom*. Cleveland: Western Reserve Geriatrics Education Center, 1989.

Raskova, Jana, Martin, Eugene G., and Shea, Stephen M. "A Second–Year Pathology Course that Emphasizes Independent Learning." *The Journal of Medical Education* 63(6): 486–488, 1988.

Ratner, Joseph, editor. *Intellegence in the Modern World: John Dewey's Philosophy*. New York: Random House, 1939.

Ratzan, Richard M. "On Teaching." *The New England of Medicine* 306(23): p.1420–1422, 1982.

Reichsman, Franz, Browning, Francis E., and Hinshaw, J. Raymond. "Observations of Undergraduate Clinical Teaching in Action." *Journal of Medical Education* 39(2): 147–163, 1964.

Reid, John D.S. and Vestrup, Judith A. "Use of a Simulation to Teach Central Venous Access." *The Journal of Medical Education* 63(3): 196–197, 1988.

Reif, Rita. "Connoisseurship in Windsor Chairs." *The New York Times*: March 28, 1982.

Riessman, Frank. "The 'Helper–Therapy' Principle." *Social Work* 10(2): 27–32, 1965.

Riley, Merle W. "Reducing 'Information Overload' in the Teaching of Pharmacology: The '200 Drug List.' " *The Journal of Medical Education* 59(6): 508–511, 1984.

Rippey, Robert M. *The Evaluation of Teaching in Medical Schools*. New York: Springer Publishing Company, 1981.

Rockoff, Mark A. "Interactions between Medical Students and Nursing Personnel." *The Journal of Medical Education* 48(8): 725–731, 1973.

Rogers, Carl. *Freedom to Learn*. Columbus, OH: Merrill Publishing Company, 1969.

Rogers, David E. "Some Musings on Medical Education: Is It Going Astray?" *Pharos* Spring: 11–14, 1982.

Rosenberg, Donna A. and Silver, Henry K. "Medical Student Abuse: An Unnecessary and Preventable Cause of Stress." *Journal of the American Medical Association* 251(6): 739–742, 1984.

Roszak, Theodore. *The Cult of Information: The Folklore of Computers and the True Art of Thinking*. New York: Pantheon Books, 1986.

Rowe, Mary B. "Wait Time and Rewards as Instructional Variables, Their Influence on Language, Logic, and Rate Control: Part 1—Wait Time." *Journal of Research on Science Teaching* 11:81–94, 1974.

Russell, I. Jon *et al.* "Effects of Three Types of Lecture Notes on Medical Student Achievement." *The Journal of Medical Education* 58(8): 627–636, 1983.

Russell, I. Jon, Hendricson, William D., and Herbert, Robert J. "Effects of Lecture Density on Medical Student Achievement." *The Journal of Medical Education* 59(11): 881–889, 1984.

Russell, John. *The New York Times*: H33, April 16, 1989.

Rutman, Leonard. *Planning Useful Evaluations*. Beverly Hills: Sage Publications, 1980.

Saffran, Murray and Yeasting, Richard A. "A First–Year,.Student–Managed Course to Correlate Basic Sciences with Clinical Medicine." *The Journal of Medical Education* 60(10): 793–797, 1985.

Sapira, Jospeh D. "A Modest Proposal: Board Certification for Medical Educators (or Quis Custodiet Ipsos Custodes?)." *Southern Medical Journal* 79(9): 1141–1141, 1986.

Sapolsky, Robert M. "Stress in the Wild." *Scientific American*: 116–122, January 1990.

Saul, Mark E. "Where Bad Teaching Is Being Taught." *The New York Times*: April 3, 1988.

Scarpinato, Len and Whitman, Neal. "Failure of the Three Minute Lecture to Result in 24 Hour Retention of Medical Facts." *Clinical Research* 38(2): 733A, 1990.

Scherger, Joseph. "A Medical Student's Perspective on Preceptors in Family Medicine." *The Journal of Family Practice* 2(3): 201–203, 1975.

Schiffman, Fred J. "The Teaching House Officer." *The Yale Journal of Biology and Medicine* 59: 55–61, 1986.

Schön, Donald A. *Educating the Reflective Practitioner.* San Francisco: Jossey–Bass Publishers, 1987.

Schwartz, William. "Education in the Classroom." *Journal of Higher Education* 51(3): 235–254, 1980

Schwenk, Thomas L. and Whitman, Neal. *Residents as Teachers: A Guide to Educational Practice.* Salt Lake City: University of Utah School of Medicine, 1984.

Schwenk, Thomas L. and Whitman, Neal. *The Physician as Teacher.* Baltimore: Williams and Wilkins, 1987.

Scriven, Michael. *The Methodology of Evaluation: Perspective of Curriculum Evaluation.* Chicago: Rand McNally, 1967.

Segal, Robert A. "What Is Good Teaching? And Why Is There So Little of It?" *The Chronicle of Higher Education*: September 24, 1979.

Seldin, Peter. "Evaluating Teaching Performance: Answers to Common Questions." *AAHE Bulletin* 40: 10, 1987.

Selye, Hans. "A Syndrome Produced by Diverse Nocuous Agents." *Nature* 138: 32, 1936.

Sheehan, T. Joseph *et al.* "Teaching Humanistic Behavior." *Teaching and Learning in Medicine* 1(2): 82–84, 1989.

Sheets, Kent J. "Teaching Skill Improvement for Graduate Medical Trainees." *Evaluation and Health Professions*: Spring 1988.

Siegler, Mark *et al.* "Effect of Role–Model Clinicians on Students' Attitudes in a Second–Year Course on Introduction to the Patient." *The Journal of Medical Education* 62(11): 935–937, 1987.

Silver, Henry.K. "Medical Students and Medical School." *Journal of the American Medical Association* 247(3): 309–310, 1982.

Sisson, J.C. "Negligence at the Bedside: Academic Malpractice." *The University of Michigan Medical Center Journal* 42: 145–146, 1976.

Skeff, Kelley *et al.* "Assessment by Attending Physicians of a Seminar Method to Improve Clinical Teaching." *The Journal of Medical Education* 59(12): 944–950, 1984.

Skinner, B.F. *Walden Two*. New York: Macmillan Company, 1948.

Smith, Lloyd. "Medical Education for the 21st Century." *The Journal of Medical Education* 60(2): 106–112, 1985.

Sophocles, Ari Jr. "Family Medicine: The Breckenridge Perspective." *Utah Medical Association Bulletin* 35(7): 12–14, 1987.

Stein, Morris. *Stimulating Creativity: Volume I. Individual Procedures.* New York: Academic Press, 1974.

Stein, Morris. *Stimulating Creativity: Volume 2. Group Procedures.* New York: Academic Press, 1975.

Stillman, Paula L. *et al.* "Effect of Immediate Student Evaluations on a Multi–Instructor Course." *The Journal of Medical Education* 58(3): 172–178, 1983.

Stillman, Paula L. *et al.* "Patient Instructors as Teachers and Evaluators." *The Journal of Medical Education* 55(3): 186–193, 1980.

Stone, John. "A Pointilist Painting." *The New York Times Magazine*, Part 2: 60, 77, October 8, 1989.

Stritter, Frank. "Faculty Evaluation and Development." In *Handbook of Health Professions Education*, edited by C.H. McGuire. San Francisco: Jossey–Bass Publishers, 1983.

Stritter, Frank. "The Learning Vector: A Developmental Approach to Clinical Instruction." *Family Practice Faculty Development Newsletter of Texas* 7(1): 1–4, 1986.

Stritter, Frank, Hain, Jack D., Grimes, David A. "Clinical Teaching Reexamined." *Journal of Medical Education* 50: 876–882, 1975.

Stuart, John and Rutherford, R.J.D. "Medical Student Concentration during Lectures." *The Lancet* No. 8088: 514–516, September 2, 1978.

Stuart, Marian R. and Lieberman, Joseph A., III. *The Fifteen–Minute Hour: Applied Psychotherapy for the Primary Care Physician.* New York: Praeger Press, 1986.

Swanson, David B. "Computer–Assisted Instruction in Health Professions Education: Promises, Prospects, and Problems." presented at the Annual Meeting of the American Academy for Cerebral Palsey and Developmental Medicine, Washington, D.C., October 24, 1984.

Swanson, R.S. *et al.* "Emergency Intravenous Access through the Femoral Vein." *Annals of Emergency Medicine* 13: 244–247, 1984.

Thomas, Lewis. "The Art of Teaching Science." *The New York Times Magazine*: March 14, 1982.

Tiberius, Richard G. *et al.* "The Use of Student Evaluative Feedback on the Improvement of Clinical Teaching." *The Journal of Higher Education* 60(6): 665–681, 1989.

Trevino, Fernando M. and Eiland, Jr., D.C. "Evaluation of a Basic Science Peer Tutorial Program for First– and Second–Year Medical Students." *Journal of Medical Education* 55(11): 952–953, 1980.

Tosteson, Daniel C. "The Oliver Wendell Holmes Society: A New Pathway to General Medical Education at Harvard Medical School." In *How to Begin Reforming the Medical Curriculum*, edited by H.S. Barrows and M.J. Peters. Springfield: Southern Illinois School of Medicine.

Verby, J.E., Schaefer, M.T., and Voeks, R.S. "Learning Forestry out of the Lumberyard: A Training Alternative for Primary Care." *The Journal of the American Medical Association* 246: 645–647, 1981.

von Oech, Roger. *A Whack on the Side of the Head.* New York: Warner Books, 1983.

Voytovich, Anthony E., Rippey, Robert M., and Pratt, D.D. "Premature Conclusions in Diagnostic Reasoning." *Journal of Medical Education* 60(4): 302, 1985.

Wales, Charles E. and Stager, Robert A. *The Guided Design Approach.* Englewood Cliffs, NJ: Educational Technology Publications, 1978.

Walker–Bartnick, Leslie A., Berger, John H., and Kappelman, Murray M. "A Model for Peer Tutoring in the Medical School Setting." *Journal of Medical Education* 59(4): 309–315, 1984.

Ware, John E. and Williams, Reed. "The Dr. Fox Effect: A Study of Lecture Effectiveness and Ratings of Instruction." *The Journal of Medical Education* 50(2): 149–155, 1975.

Weinholtz, Donn. *Teaching During Attending Rounds: A Manual for Attending Physicians*. Iowa City: Office of Consultation and Research in Medical Education, University of Iowa, 1987.

Whalen, James P. "Evaluating Students." *The Journal of Medical Education* 60(7): 584, 1985.

Whitman, Neal. "Choosing and Using Methods of Teaching." *Performance and Instruction* 20(5): 16–19, 1981a.

Whitman, Neal. "Developing Lecture Skills." In *Clinical Teaching for Medical Residents: Roles, Techniques, and Programs*, edited by J.C. Edwards and R.L. Marier. New York: Springer Press, 1988.

Whitman, Neal. "Developing Teaching Skills for Medical School Faculty." *Human Pathology* 21(1): 1990.

Whitman, Neal. "Evaluating Family Practice Residency Programs: A Guide to Systematic Data Collection." *Family Medicine* 15(1): 6–10, 1983.

Whitman, Neal. "Evaluations Can Isolate Teaching from Learning." *Instructional Innovator* 26(3): 35–36, 1981b.

Whitman, Neal. "A Guide to Clinical Performance Testing." Idea Paper No. 7. Manhattan, KS: Center for Faculty Evaluation and Development, Kansas State University, 1982.

Whitman, Neal. *Peer Teaching: To Teach is to Learn Twice*. Washington, D.C.: Associaton for the Study of Higher Education, 1988.

Whitman, Neal. *There Is No Gene for Good Teaching: A Handbook on Lecturing for Medical Teachers*. Salt Lake City: University of Utah School of Medicine, 1982.

Whitman, Neal and Burgess, Paul R. "Teaching Basic Science: Dr. Fox in the Physiology Chicken Coop." *Medical Education* 22: 393–397, 1988.

Whitman, Neal and Cockayne, Thomas. *Evaluating Medical School Courses: A User–Centered Handbook*. Salt Lake City: University of Utah School of Medicine, 1984.

Whitman, Neal and Ferrey, Anthony. "Effective Medical Teaching as Characterized by Medical School Teaching Award Winners" presented at the Annual Meeting of the American Educational Research Association, San Francisco, April 16, 1986.

Whitman, Neal and Goodenough, Gerald. *Improving the Teaching of Geriatrics: An Interactive Approach for the Clinician*. Cleveland: Western Reserve Geriatrics Education Center, 1987.

Whitman, Neal and Schwenk, Thomas L. "Faculty Evaluation as a Means of Faculty Development." *The Journal of Family Practice* 14(6): 1097–1101, 1982.

Whitman, Neal and Schwenk, Thomas L. *A Handbook for Group Discussion Leaders: Alternatives to Lecturing Medical Students to Death*. Salt Lake City: University of Utah School of Medicine, 1983.

Whitman, Neal and Schwenk, Thomas L. *Preceptors as Teachers: A Guide to Clinical Teaching*. Salt Lake City: University of Utah School of Medicine, 1984.

Whitman, Neal, Spendlove, David, and Clark, Claire. *Increasing Student Learning: A Faculty Guide to Student Stress*. Washington, D.C.: Association for the Study of Higher Education, 1986.

Whitman, Neal, Spendlove, David, and Clark, Claire. *Student Stress: Effects and Solutions*. Washington, D.C.: Association for the Study of Higher Education, 1984.

Whitman, Neal and Weiss, Elaine. *Faculty Evaluation: The Use of Explicit Criteria for Promotion, Retention, and Tenure.* Washington, D.C.: American Association of Higher Education, 1982.

Whitman, Neal *et al.* "Clinical Impressions." letter to the editor, *The Journal of Medical Education* 63(2): 153, 1988.

Wilkes, Michael S. and Shuchman, Miriam. "Pitching Doctors." *The New York Times Magazine*: 88–89, 126–129, November 5, 1989.

Woods, Donald. *What is Problem Solving and Background Ideas.* The McMaster Problem Solving Program, Unit 2. Hamilton, Ontario: McMaster University, 1983.

Woolliscroft, James O. and Schwenk, Thomas L. "Teaching and Learning in the Ambulatory Setting." *Academic Medicine* 64(11): 644–648, 1989.

Wurman, Richard Saul. *Information Anxiety.* New York: Doubleday, 1989.

Yerkes, Robert M. and Dodson, J.D. "The Relationship of Strength Stimulus to Rapidity of Habit Formation." *Journal of Comparative and Neurological Psychology* 18: 459–482, 1908.

Index of Names

Editing, Design and Production by

Elaine Weiss
Educational Dimensions
Salt Lake City, Utah